Everything you always wanted to know about Marijuana*

Everything you always wanted to know about Marijuana*

*But Were Too Stoned To Ask

Tim Pilcher

ilex

An Hachette UK Company
www.hachette.co.uk

First published in the United States in 2017 by ILEX,
a division of Octopus Publishing Group Ltd.
Octopus Publishing Group, Carmelite House
50 Victoria Embankment, London, EC4Y 0DZ
www.octopusbooksusa.com

An earlier edition of this book was published as
Pilcher's Marijuana Miscellany by Ilex in 2014

Distributed in the US by Hachette Book Group
1290 Avenue of the Americas, 4th & 5th Floors,
New York, NY 10104

Distributed in Canada by Canadian Manda Group
664 Annette St., Toronto, Ontario, Canada M6S 2C8

Publisher: Roly Allen
Editorial Director: Zara Larcombe
Managing Editor: Frank Gallaugher
Editor: Rachel Silverlight
Art Director: Julie Weir
Cover Design: Ben Gardiner
Picture Research: Katie Greenwood
Production Controller: Lucy Carter

Additional text by E. M. Frost and Rachel Silverlight

ISBN: 978-1-78157-799-8

Printed and bound in the UK

10 9 8 7 6 5 4 3 2 1

"The motion picture you are
about to witness may startle you.

It would not have been possible,
otherwise, to sufficiently emphasize the
frightful toll of the new drug menace, which
is destroying the youth of America in
alarmingly increasing numbers.

Marihuana is that drug—a violent
narcotic—an unspeakable scourge.

The Real Public Enemy Number One!"

REEFER MADNESS, 1936

GATEWAY DRUG

CANNABIS HAS LONG BEEN cited as a "gateway drug" leading users on to other narcotics. This controversial theory has yet to be proved conclusively though, since while some scientific studies have shown that the consumption of cannabis can possibly predict a higher risk of subsequent use of "harder" illicit drugs, other studies show that it can't! Many studies looked at correlation, rather than causation, which is notoriously difficult to prove.

According to the US-based National Institute on Drug Abuse (NIDA), "People who abuse drugs are also likely to be cigarette smokers. More than two-thirds of drug abusers are regular tobacco smokers, a rate more than triple that of the rest of the population."

A 2011 US–Finnish twin study revealed those who started smoking tobacco by the age of 12 were 26 times more likely to start using cannabis or other illicit drugs by age 17, compared to those who never smoked. It appears that tobacco smoking and drinking are the most powerful predictors of later use of illicit drugs. So, the true "gateway drugs" may in fact be nicotine and alcohol.

But whichever camp you fall in, the debate looks likely to rage on for some time to come.

MARIJUANA SLANG

CANNABIS HAS A LANGUAGE all of its own. Smokers are referred to as Tokers, Stoners, Blazers, Space Cadets, Dope Headers, Vipers, Wasteoids, Potheads, and Herbalists, who then proceed to Skin-Up, Roll, or Get One On. After Blazing Away, they tend to be Wasted, Stoned, Mashed, Baked, Caned, Toasted, Annihilated, Gone, Blasted, Blunted, Battered, or simply just Irie. Some might get The Munchies (sudden hunger, for particularly sweet and/or salty snacks), or even Cottonmouth (lack of saliva creating a dry, parched sensation in the mouth), but what no one wants is The Whiteys (nausea and a panic attack).

———— FIVE BEST GLOBAL FESTIVALS ————

THERE ARE SEVERAL EVENTS THAT celebrate marijuana, where you can partake of a whole range of weed and mingle with other marijuana fans.

Hempfest, Seattle, Washington, USA (August) With impressive crowds sometimes reaching 310,000, this is one of the largest pro-pot events in the world, despite only launching in 1991. Speakers have included Senators, Congressmen, and actor Woody Harrelson.
www.hempfest.org

Nimbin Mardigrass, Nimbin, New South Wales, Australia (May) Full of talks and bands, this very peaceful and polite protest event draws crowds from all over the world. Despite constant run-ins with the local police the show has been running for 21 years and places a strong emphasis on fancy dress with the Ganja Fairies—"The spirit of the MardiGrass"—parade.
www.nimbinmardigrass.com

Spannabis, Barcelona, Spain (March) Attracting over 20,000 green gardeners from around the globe, this Spanish event has its own grower's competition with awards for best nutrients, tools, and growth systems.
www.spannabis.com

The High Times Cannabis Cup, throughout the USA (dates vary) The original Cannabis Cup was held every November in Amsterdam, The Netherlands, from 1988 until the event was shut down in 2014. Thankfully the US Cannabis Cup, first held in Denver, Colorado in 2012, is still going strong and expanding into new locations every year.
www.cannabiscup.com

Cannafest, Prague, Czech Republic (November) Founded in 2010, Prague's international cannabis tradeshow has grown every year. Exhibits cover every angle from cannabis technology and cultivation, to activism and enjoyment.

> "They lie about marijuana. Tell you pot-smoking makes you unmotivated. Lie! When you're high, you can do everything you normally do, just as well. You just realize that it's not worth the fucking effort. There is a difference."
>
> BILL HICKS, *American comedian* (1961–1994)

TOP FIVE STONER FLICKS

O F COURSE, IT PROBABLY HELPS to smoke a bowl before watching any of these:

Up in Smoke (DIR. LOU ADLER, 1978) The legendary, original, and best stoner movie of all time sees Cheech Marin and Tommy Chong get deported to Mexico and then, unwittingly, drive a van made entirely of grass back over the border to perform at the "Battle of the Bands" in L.A. while being pursued by incompetent DEA officers. This film paved the way for the buddy stoner comedy genre.

Dazed & Confused (DIR. RICHARD LINKLATER, 1993) Richaed Linklater's cult coming-of-age comedy follows a group of incoming seniors and freshmen on the last day of school in 1976—and everyone's trying to get drunk, stoned, or both. With a killer soundtrack and great ensemble cast, this is an absolute classic of the stoner genre that evokes the mad, desperate freedom of when school's out for the summer.

Friday (DIR. F. GARY GRAY, 1995) Smokey (Chris Tucker) and recently fired Craig (Ice Cube) are a couple of homies getting stoned on a dealer's weed and watching their neighbors' antics in South Central L.A. The pair find themselves in trouble when they have to pay the dealer the $200 for the stash they lit up.

Dude, Where's My Car? (DIR. DANNY LEINER, 2000) Jesse (Ashton Kutcher) and Chester (Seann William Scott) are two bumbling potheads who can't remember where they left their car after a night of hard-core partying. They embark on a quest to find out what happened the previous night. They meet their angry girlfriends, whose house they trashed, an angry street gang, a transsexual stripper, and a group of aliens in human form. This film is the template for *The Hangover* (2009), and was directed by Danny Leiner, who went on to direct *Harold and Kumar go to White Castle* (2004).

Pineapple Express (DIR. DAVID GORDON GREEN, 2008) This very funny action/comedy sees stoner and process server Dale Denton (Seth Rogen) and his cannabis dealer Saul Silver (James Franco) on the run from cops and hit men when Denton witnesses Silver's boss killed. The title refers to a particularly rare strain of weed, "It's, like, the rarest. It's almost a shame to smoke it. It's like killing a unicorn. With, like, a bomb." And there are heaps of other stoner jokes throughout.

ETYMOLOGY: BONG (NOUN)

A water pipe for smoking marijuana through. Like a Shisha or Hookah Pipe, the water cools the smoke down, making it more pleasant to inhale. The term comes from Vietnam War veterans, who returned to the US with the Thai phrase, *baung*, literally meaning "cylindrical wooden tube." Soldiers even smoked weed through the barrel of their rifles.

------ HENRY FORD'S MARIJUANA MOBILE ------

MOTORCAR ENGINEER and entrepreneur Henry Ford was constantly pushing the frontiers of technology. In 1925 he told the *New York Times* that ethyl alcohol was "the fuel of the future," believing that grain alcohol derived from crops such as soybean and hemp would resolve any energy crisis. "Why use up the forests which were centuries in the making, and the mines, which required ages to lay down," he queried, "if we can get the equivalent of forest and mineral products in the annual growth of the fields?" He also foresaw that plastics would be the building material of tomorrow.

In the December 1941 issue of *Popular Mechanics* he revealed a new type of car made from blended cellulose bioplastics, derived from flax, wheat, spruce and, yup, you guessed it, hemp. The last ingredient's fiber was also used as a strengthener. Ford's vision was to "grow automobiles from the soil." The car's bodywork was supposedly ten times stronger than steel and 30 percent lighter. Ford's vision saw the benefits of hemp, both as a construction material and as a fuel, but in the 12 years it took to develop his car, the political landscape had changed, and the plant had gone from potential savior for US agriculture to vilified "Demon Weed." His experimental car never made it to the production lines, but it was the inspiration to Cheech and Chong's van made out of marijuana in their film, *Up in Smoke.*

------ BONGS ------

FIRST BROUGHT BACK FROM the Far East by Vietnam War veterans, the bong is one of the more fun ways to communally share some smoke. These contraptions involve burning a small piece of hash or grass in a bowl that sits on a narrow stalk, which is inserted into a large chamber, from where the rising smoke is inhaled.

Today, bongs come in all shapes and sizes, and you can buy ones that look like guns, ones that have water or ice cube chambers in them for a cool smoke, and even ones shaped like an alien's head with four mouthpieces, so you can all toke together.

Creativity is a key element of "bong culture" with stoners making them out of practically anything they can get their hands on, from hollowed-out fruit, Tupperware, old Nintendos, and Christmas decorations. As actor/comedian Denis Leary joked, "Remember that friend in High School, who wanted to make bongs out of everything? Making bongs out of apples and oranges and shit. One day you find your friend going 'Hey look, man, I made a bong out of my HEAD! Put the pot in this ear and suck it out of this one, go on take a hit!'"

—— "STOP THIS MURDEROUS SMOKE" ——

ON OCTOBER 16, 1933, a 21-year-old man, Victor Licata, killed his entire family of five—including the pet dog—with an axe in Tampa, Florida. The case became a cause célèbre, with the newspapers quickly blaming Licata's pot smoking as the reason for his violent rampage, with sensational, inflammatory headlines like, "Marijuana Maniac!"

The *Tampa Morning Tribune* stated in its story that "…It may or may not be wholly true that the pernicious marijuana cigarette is responsible for the murderous mania of a Tampa young man in exterminating all the members of his family within his reach—but

whether or not the poisonous mind-wrecking weed is mainly accountable for the tragedy, its sale should not be, and should never have been, permitted here or elsewhere." Even the police clearly doubted that the cannabis was the cause of Licata's horrendous actions, but nevertheless, the case was quickly picked up by well known prohibitionists like Harry J. Anslinger, the head of the newly-formed Federal Bureau of Narcotics, who cited it in order to ease the passage of the 1937 Marijuana Tax Act, which effectively outlawed weed in the USA.

In fact, Victor Licata suffered from a form of early on-set dementia ("dementia praecox with homicidal tendencies"), and marijuana was not mentioned in any psychiatric reports. He eventually hanged himself in the Florida State Hospital on December 4, 1950.

Licata's story was the inspiration behind Cornell Woolrich's (AKA William Irish) 1941 pulp novel, *Marihuana*, and it was mentioned in the 1936 propaganda film, *Tell Your Children* (AKA *Reefer Madness*): "Yes. I remember. Just a young boy…under the influence of drugs…who killed his entire family with an axe."

—"HE HID IT IN THE ONE PLACE HE KNEW— HE COULD HIDE SOMETHING: HIS ASS."

WHEN CHRISTOPHER WALKEN UTTERS this immortal line in *Pulp Fiction* (1994) he's talking about his war buddy's gold watch, but such a quote could easily refer to any seasoned—or amateur—drug smuggler today. Shoving anything up your ass for the purposes of storage and/or transport could be considered pretty near the top of the wrongness scale, but when it comes to drug smuggling, the Anal Express is just the tip of the shitberg. Here are a few of the more bizarre and sometimes ingenious ways people have tried to smuggle marijuana across country lines:

In early 2013, police in Mexicali, Mexico, confiscated a cannon made out of PVC piping that was used to volley packages of marijuana across a fence into California. Its ammunition caliber was about 13 kilograms. Catapults and T-shirt cannons have also been used to air-drop weed across surprisingly large distances.

Not sure what to do with your old, obsolete games console? Why not re-enact a 2010 attempt to smuggle marijuana into New Jersey using a hollowed-out Nintendo Wii. Try to be successful this time.

Drug smugglers clearly have no respect for the dead, as evidenced by a man in Dallas who was stopped by police for running a red light and turned out to be hiding 100 pounds of marijuana in a casket in the back of his van. Luckily there was no room left for a corpse.

In May 2013 El Paso, Texas, customs workers discovered 591 pounds of marijuana stuffed into plaster figurines imported from Mexico.

At JFK airport in 2006, authorities confiscated twelve bricks of marijuana from persons unknown. Upon further inspection, it was found that the marijuana bricks were actually being used to smuggle a smaller shipment of hashish. (Apparently this ruse is sometimes used by kingpins further up the ladder in order to trick drug smuggling organizations further down the assembly line into thinking they're moving cheaper merchandise, so they'll charge less.)

While the above point at least makes business sense, this one makes no sense at all: The Drug Enforcement Administration once apprehended a traveler attempting to smuggle three bullets into Andrade, California…inside a package of weed.

In August 2013 the US Border Patrol caught a scuba diver attempting to smuggle eight pounds of herb into the country from Canada by swimming almost a mile across the St. Clair River into Michigan. This man gets extra credit for fitness and determination, if not success.

MEDICAL MARIJUANA:
WHAT'S THE SCORE?

OVER THE LAST FEW DECADES, the medical use of marijuana has been steadily gaining ground and is now decriminalized in a number of states. But cannabis has been enjoyed for its medical properties for thousands of years, going back to Ancient China where hemp seed was used as a food source. These days marijuana is known to be effective in treating a great number and variety of conditions including Alzheimer's disease, arthritis, cancer, depression, HIV/AIDS, insomnia, multiple sclerosis (MS), and others. It almost sounds too good to be true—what is it in marijuana that makes it so damn good?

The answer is cannabinoids, the chemical compounds occurring in cannabis, in particular CBD and THC (although it's very likely we'll be discovering benefits in lesser-known cannabinoids as medical marijuana becomes increasingly accepted and more research is done). Cannabinoids mimic the effects of the naturally occurring compounds that work with the "endocannabinoid system," which all mammals have, which work help regulate the body, keeping imbalances in check and minimizing pain and damage throughout the body.

> "Is marijuana addictive? Yes, in the sense that most of the really pleasant things in life are worth endlessly repeating."
> RICHARD NEVILLE, *Writer and Co-editor of* Oz *magazine (1941–2016)*

WHAT'S IN A NAME?

CANNABIS HAS QUITE POSSIBLY MORE monikers than any other drug. Some relate to its appearance, like "Tea," or a particular strain or the location where it's grown, like "Maui Wowie." Others refer to the way of smoking it, like "Blunt" or "Bowl" (as in the bowl of a smoking pipe). It has also gone under all of these names at some point or other: Pot, Grass, Weed, Smoke, Reefer, Mezz, Herb, Bush, Green, Mary Jane, MJ, Chronic, Spliff, Joint, Ganja, Sensei, Sinsemilla, Bud, Hemp, Dope, Draw, Kush, Hydro, Skunk, Thai Stick, Charas, Charge, Black, Hash, Hashish, Kif, Purple Haze, White Widow, Roach, Soap Bar, Bongo, Cheeba, Dagga, Diesel, Shit, Hemp, Muggles, Solid, Wacky Baccy, Gage, Stash, Sweet Leaf, and many, many more!

MULTI-CHOC-CHIP KOMA KOOKIES

BROWNIES AND COOKIES ARE THE mainstay of cannabis cooking. However, these are the best—light, soft, chewy and chocolaty, and very moorish. This recipe makes 12 large cookies.

1 cup/250g cannabutter (see page 73)	1/2 tsp baking soda
2/3 cup/125g white sugar	1/2 tsp salt
2/3 cup/125g brown granulated sugar	1 small milk chocolate bar or chips
1 large egg	1 small dark chocolate bar or chips
1 tsp vanilla extract	1 small white chocolate bar or chips
2 cups/280g plain flour	

Instructions:

1 Blend the cannabutter and sugars together in a bowl.

2 Beat the egg in and add the vanilla.

3 Sift the flour, baking soda, and salt in and fold into the mixture.

4 Break up the chocolate bars and sprinkle and mix them in.

5 Spread the cookie dough on a greased baking sheet and bake for around 8–10 minutes at 375F/190C.

6 Cut the baked dough into required sizes. Best served slightly warm.

THE HORROR OF WEED

A SPATE OF HORROR FILMS in the late seventies and eighties equated drug use—particularly marijuana as the teenage drug of choice—and general immorality with certain and horrible death. Horror filmmakers in the late nineties and early twenty-first century then took up that mantle and continued the cannabis carnage. Here are some of the movies that you're most likely to get murdered in, or at the very least be forced to watch all your friends die, if you're a stoner, :

HALLOWEEN (1978)

MOST OF THE FRIDAY THE 13TH
FRANCHISE (1980–2003)

FRIDAY THE 13TH (2009 REBOOT)

POLTERGEIST (1982)

SHROOMS (2007)

SLEEPAWAY CAMP (1983)

SLEEPAWAY CAMP II: UNHAPPY
CAMPERS (1988)

THE THING (1982)

THE DEVIL'S REJECTS (2005)

ZOMBIELAND (2009)

CABIN FEVER (2002)

IDLE HANDS (1999)

LAST HOUSE ON THE LEFT (1972
AND THE 2009 REMAKE)

FREDDY'S DEAD: THE FINAL
NIGHTMARE (1991)

FINAL DESTINATION 2 (2003)

THE CABIN IN THE WOODS (2012)

HOT KNIFING

ALSO KNOWN AS "SPOTS" OR "BLADES," this method of smoking hash is a slightly sketchy forerunner to the (also slightly sketchy) dab method. While diminishing in popularity in New Zealand and the UK—and virtually unknown in the USA—hot-knifing involves heating up two large flat knives, squashing a lump of hash between them, and inhaling the rising smoke. To help funnel the smoke a bottomless glass or plastic bottle (known as a "Spottle" or "Hooter") is used. Often this is frozen to provide a cooler smoke. In 2008, six New Zealand soldiers stationed in Afghanistan were sent home in disgrace after "Spotting" hash, using a soldering iron!

HEROES OF HEMP:
BOB DYLAN & THE BEATLES

BOB DYLAN WAS ALWAYS A STONER and was high when he recorded the 1966 track *Rainy Day Women #12 & 35* on his *Blonde on Blonde* album. The song was banned from many radio stations because of its pro-pot chorus, "But I would not feel so all alone, Everybody must get stoned."

Dylan was also responsible for switching The Beatles on to weed on August 28, 1964 at New York's Delmonico Hotel. Although George Harrison recalled The Beatles' initial encounter with cannabis, in 1960, wasn't so great: "We first got marijuana from an older drummer with another group in Liverpool. We didn't actually try it until after we'd been to Hamburg…Everybody was saying, 'This stuff isn't doing anything.'"

But Dylan's shit was on the level and The Beatles' manager, Brian Epstein, kept saying, "I'm so high I'm on the ceiling. I'm up on the ceiling." "That, for me, was the first time I smoked marijuana. And I laughed, and I laughed, and I laughed," Ringo Starr recalled.

John Lennon said, "I don't remember much what we talked about. We were smoking dope, drinking wine, and generally being rock 'n' rollers and having a laugh, you know, and surrealism. It was party time." Paul McCartney admitted that day had a profound effect on The Beatles' music, to the point that by 1969 they were singing, "Smoke pot, smoke pot, everybody smoke pot" at the end of *I Am the Walrus*.

SINSEMILLA LADY

THIS DELICIOUS AND REFRESH-ING green cocktail is sure to get the party started. First you need to make a tincture using tequila (see page 51).

15ml (1/2fl oz.) of tequila/cannabis tincture
30ml (1fl oz.) of melon liqueur
90ml (3fl oz.) of grapefruit juice
slice of melon
slice of lime
2 cherries
crushed ice

Put all of the key ingredients—the melon liqueur, tincture, grapefruit juice, and ice—into a shaker and shake vigorously. Pour the concoction into a highball glass of your choice and garnish with the melon, lime, and cherries.

INDIAN BHANG

INDIA HAS A LONG TRADITION involving cannabis. It's said that Buddha himself survived for six years by living solely on hemp seeds. Many Hindu sadhus (holy men) use cannabis, known as bhang, as a sacrament, like Rastafarians, on religious days such as the Holi festival, and to induce transcendental states.

While sadhus do smoke grass in clay pipe "chillums" many Indians and Nepalese prefer to consume cannabis by imbibing it in a drink called Bhang Ki Thandai or Sardai. This is a bit like a weed-infused lassi made with almonds, spices, milk, and sugar. The female plant and other ingredients are ground down into a paste and then boiled with milk to extract the active THC element, which is then sieved and

drunk cold. Cannabis is legal to grow and sell in India, with a permit, and is often preferred on the sub-continent to alcohol.

SMOKING ETIQUETTE

NO ONE WANTS TO BE A DRAG when sharing a joint, so here's some polite rules on how not to be rude. Generally, the person rolling blazes up first. Don't take forever skinning up, people get impatient. If you get into difficulty ask for help. Take two tokes and pass to the left, is generally the polite way to smoke in a group. Whatever you do, don't Bogart that joint! That is, don't hang onto it for ages before passing it on—take your tokes and share the wealth. Don't drool on the end of the joint, no one likes a soggy roach!

> "When I was promoting *Green Hornet*, Sony asked me to not tell too many weed stories. And I said, 'I don't think I'm capable of doing that.' It's kind of the only thing I can talk about."
>
> SETH ROGEN, *Actor and Writer (b. 1982)*

FIVE OF THE BEST AMSTERDAM COFFEE SHOPS

AMSTERDAM IS NOTORIOUS FOR ITS "Coffee shops" where you can order some supreme green to go with your latte. Different cafes stock different strains of grass and hash, either pre-rolled or DIY. Here are some of the most famous cafes, but there are plenty more off the beaten track that have fewer tokin' tourists.

DampKring Made famous by a guest appearance in *Ocean's Twelve* (2004), this is one of the more traditional smoking dens with psychedelic art on the walls and a friendly atmosphere.

The Bulldog Admittedly the most touristy of all the cafes, but still has a good atmosphere. Originally starting in a small basement, there are now five branches across the city. Also has a five-star hostel to crash in when it all gets too much.

The Grasshopper Four floors of flaming fun, this venue not only has the essential coffee shop, but also pubs and restaurants, meaning you need never leave. All lit-up in green at night it was name-checked in The Streets' song about getting wasted in Amsterdam, *Too Much Brandy*.

Barney's Recently renovated, this 23-year-old institution is now a hi-tech cafe with each table sporting a digital menu and vaporizer. It's also the home to incredible milkshakes and seven Cannabis Cup Winners, so you know the quality is good! Up by the Centraal Station, it opens at 7am. How much weed can you smoke in 18 hours before it closes again?

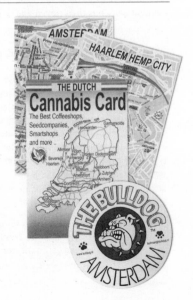

Grey Area This tiny shop boasts some great strains and a celebrity clientele, but other than that it's worth mentioning just because it's basically right next door to the Amsterdam Duck Store. That's right.

——— HERO OF HEMP: SETH ROGEN ———

PROBABLY ONE OF THE MOST SUCCESSFUL stoners that Hollywood has ever known, actor/writer/producer/director/comedian Seth Rogen is a household name.

As a filmmaker, Rogen has made stoner movies not only acceptable, but massive money-making enterprises: witness *Pineapple Express* (2008), *This Is the End* (2013), *50/50* (2011), *Superbad* (2007), and *Knocked Up* (2007). As an actor, he most often plays the loveable stoner, and he does it extremely well—most likely a result of the research he's been doing for the role his whole life. Instead of shying away from pot's place in his creative process, he's always been very honest about using the drug as a creative tool: "I smoke a lot of weed when I write, generally speaking," said Seth Rogen to HighRoulette.com in 2013. "I don't know if it helps me write. It makes me not mind that I'm writing. And I don't know if it makes me work better, but it makes me not care that I'm working. Who wants to work? But if you're stoned, it doesn't seem like work."

——————— HIGH TIMES ———————

FOUNDED IN 1974 by activist and pioneering underground journalist Thomas King Forcade, *High Times* is a US counterculture magazine that celebrates all manner of illicit highs. Forcade was an underground journalist, activist, and drug smuggler, and this latter role provided the title's financial backing. The erratic Forcade often pitted staff against each other and once even fired the entire team, rehiring them all the next day. The magazine hit a zeitgeist and in just four years had reached a circulation of 420,000 (rivalling *Rolling Stone* and *National Lampoon*) when Forcade committed suicide in 1978. His lawyer friend Michael Kennedy picked up the reins and shifted the magazine's focus away from LSD, mushrooms, and cocaine, and on to marijuana.

It soon became synonymous with sinsemilla, starting the infamous Cannabis Cup in Amsterdam—which was established by Steve Hager in 1987, who was then made Editor-in-Chief of the publication the following year. Since then the magazine has branched out into a number of other awards, as well as festivals, filmmaking, book publishing and even a compilation album of Herbal Hip-Hop songs (*High Times Presents THC Vol. 1*). 2007 even saw a controversial reality TV series, *High Times Office*.

The magazine itself has featured a roster of impressive contributors including authors Charles Bukowski, Truman Capote, Samuel R. Delany, and Hunter S. Thompson, cannabis activist Ed Rosenthal, and reggae star Peter Tosh.

SHE TRADED HER BODY FOR DRUGS— AND KICKS!

Marijuana Girl

N. R. DeMexico

B328
35¢
K

NEVER WAS THERE SO OUTSPOKEN A NOVEL AS THIS... TELLING THE PLAIN, UNCENSORED TRUTH ABOUT TEEN-AGE ADDICTS — AND THEIR DESPERATE SEARCH FOR THRILLS!

HIGHS & LOWS OF THE

ROAD TO LEGALIZATION

THE RE-LEGALIZATION OF MARIJUANA has been a long time coming; and with weed still illegal under federal law and its consumption still largely demonized by conservatives and denied by most politicians and other authorities, there's still a ways to go. But the times they are a changin'. Cannabis is now legal for medical use in most states, and in 2012 Colorado and Washington were the first states to legalize it for recreational use, signalling that high times may indeed be upon us.

1911: Massachusetts becomes the first state to ban cannabis

1936: Release of anti-marijuana propaganda film, Reefer Madness

1937: Marihuana Tax Act is passed, enforced by the Narcotics Bureau

1941: Industrial hemp production temporarily encouraged to help with the war effort

1943: Medical products containing or derived from cannabis are removed

1945: All hemp production, subsidized during the war, is re-banned
The LaGuardia Report finds that smoking marijuana does not lead to addiction

1965: The pro-marijuana counter-culture movement breaks into public consciousness as the first organized protests against the prohibition of cannabis, convened by Beat poet Allen Ginsberg, take place

1969–70: Cannabis-law-reformation group Amorphia is founded in California, followed by NORML in Washington, D.C.

1970: Cannabis is classified as a Schedule 1 drug carrying the highest penalties for possession, sale, and cultivation, under the new Controlled Substances Act

1972: The Schafer Commission recommends cannabis be decriminalized for personal use.
President Nixon rejects the recommendation.

1973: Oregon reduces penalties for possession of marijuana

1975: President Jimmy Carter endorses the Schafer Commission's finding and recommends the decriminalization of cannabis for adults.

1980: Ronald Reagan becomes president, ending an era of relaxation of attitudes toward marijuana under Jimmy Carter, and institutes the "War on Drugs."

1986: The Antidrug Abuse Act of 1986 is passed by Congress, ushering in mandatory minimum sentences for even low-level abuses

1988: The Antidrug Abuse Amendments Act brings in life sentences for offenders with two or more prior convictions

1991: San Francisco passes a popular ordinance to allow patients access to medical marijuana

1996: California becomes the first state to legalize medical marijuana

1998: Alaska, Arizona, Oregon, and Washington states pass laws to allow medical use of cannabis, beginning a wave of marijuana-law relaxation across many more states, over several years to the present day

2005: The Federal Ban on marijuana is upheld by the Supreme Court, making marijuana a prohibited substance even in the 11 states that permitted it at the time

2010: California votes against the legalization of marijuana for recreational use

2012: Colorado and Washington become the first states to legalize small amounts of marijuana for personal recreational use

2013: U.S. Justice Department announces that it will not interfere with state laws legalizing marijuana, and the DEA will only act where offences involve firearms, violence, distribution to states where marijuana is still illegal, or where profits fund organized crime

2014: Justice Department recommends Native Americans on reservations should be allowed to grow and sell marijuana even in states where it is illegal

2020: At the time of writing, marijuana has been legalized for medical purposes in 33 states and Washington D.C., and is legal for recreational purposes in 11, along with the capital. Meanwhile, high-less CBD products are taking the world by storm. Watch this space

---

——— ETYMOLOGY: MARIJUANA (NOUN) ———

The actual etymological origins of the word marijuana stem from the Mexican Spanish *marihuana*, but before that the trail goes cold. Some have postulated that it comes from the Spanish proper name *Maria Juana* or "Mary Jane," but, no one really knows why the name and the plant came to be associated.

WEED DREAMS

MANY REGULAR CANNABIS CONSUMERS report that they 'don't dream' when they're blazed, and after a couple of days off the smoke, back come the dreams – often with an added dose of surrealness. But are we actually experiencing fewer dreams? Or is our stoned sleep just so good and deep that we don't remember our dreams when we wake up?

Dreaming takes place during the REM (rapid eye movement) phase of our sleep cycle, which lasts for up to two hours every night. Various studies have suggested that THC can suppress REM sleep, meaning that users of high-THC strains of weed might not have enough time to get into their dreams properly. On the other hand, CBD has been reported to increase the duration and quality of REM sleep, which means longer and better dreams.

While we don't know a great deal about dreaming, scientists believe that REM sleep is an essential function for our bodies, helping us to process daily trauma and necessary for the proper functioning of our memory. We don't know for sure that THC impairs our REM sleep—and insomnia sufferers will probably agree that not getting all your REM sleep is better than not getting any sleep—but it's probably worth having a few nights off once in a while!

> "There was no time to weigh chances. There was no such thing as chances anyway, in the distorted perspective of the weed fumes."
>
> CORNELL WOOLRICH, *Marihuana (1941)*

WHO INHALED?

WHAT'S WITH POLITICIANS CONFESSING they tried marijuana in their reckless youth … but they didn't inhale and they didn't like it anyway!? But you might be surprised by which famous statesmen and women freely admit having used it. Heck, some of them even enjoyed it! Why not test your knowledge on the "Who inhaled" quiz?

1. **Bill Clinton**
2. **Barack Obama**
3. **Sarah Palin**
4. **Arnold Schwarzenegger**
5. **George W. Bush**
6. **Al Gore**
7. **Bernie Sanders**
8. **George Washington & Thomas Jefferson**
9. **John F. Kennedy**
10. **Donald Trump**

1. NO: "DIDN'T LIKE IT, DIDN'T INHALE, AND NEVER TRIED IT AGAIN" 2. YES: "WHEN I WAS A KID, I INHALED, FREQUENTLY, THAT WAS THE POINT." 3. YES: ADMITTED USING IT "IN THE PAST." 4. FAMOUSLY SMOKED MARIJUANA IN 1977 DOCUMENTARY PUMPING IRON: "I DID SMOKE A JOINT AND I DID INHALE." BUT CLAIMS HE HASN'T TAKEN IT SINCE THE '70S. 5. YES—HE EVENTUALLY ADMITTED "I DON'T WANT SOME LITTLE KID DOING WHAT I TRIED." 6. YES. AL GORE IS KNOWN TO HAVE SMOKED WEED AFTER RETURNING FROM VIETNAM IN 1971, BUT CLAIMED HIS USE WAS "INFREQUENT AND RARE." 7. YES, AND HE "COUGHED A LOT." 8. POSSIBLY. THE FOUNDING FATHERS WERE CERTAINLY EARLY ADVOCATES OF THE CROP KNOWN AS HEMP—BUT PROBABLY MORE FOR ITS USE IN PRODUCTS SUCH AS CLOTHING AND PAPER RATHER THAN ITS PSYCHOACTIVE PROPERTIES. 9. OH HELL YES! WHETHER FOR RECREATIONAL USE OR MEDICINAL, FOR RELIEF FROM HIS CHRONIC BACK, IS NOT KNOWN. 10. NOPE. THE 45TH PRESIDENT OF THE UNITED STATES CLAIMS TO HAVE NEVER CONSUMED ALCOHOL, CIGARETTES, OR RECREATIONAL DRUGS.

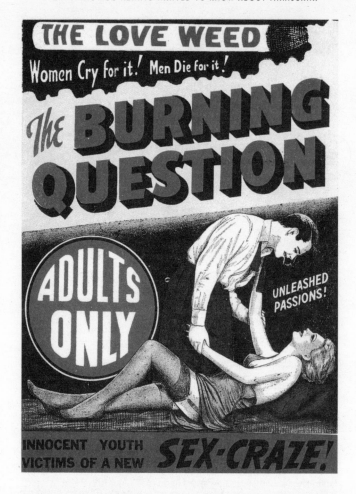

ETYMOLOGY: DAGGA (NOUN)

South African term for Cannabis Indicia and Sativa. Derived from Afrikaans and the Hottentot word, *dachab*, circa 1670–1675.

> "Weed's not as bad as everything else, cause weed is a background substance. You know what I mean, you can smoke some herb and still function. You ain't crisp…but you'll function."
>
> DAVE CHAPPELLE, *Comedian (b. 1973)*

POISON!

MARIJUANA HAS HAD A LONG and troubled history with respect to the law, most often because it's been automatically equated with far more addictive and destructive drugs such as opium, cocaine, and meth, as well as it being habitually mislabeled as a narcotic.

In the early 1920s, Egypt was experiencing a significant hashish problem among its population, and prevailed upon the League of Nations to criminalize the drug and help slow international traffic. The Egyptian delegate at the 1925 Geneva Opium Convention called hashish "a dangerous narcotic" and "more harmful than opium," and asserted that most lunatics in Egyptian asylums were hashish abusers. He asked for global controls prohibiting the import/export of cannabis, or Indian Hemp, and cannabis was duly sanctioned alongside opium and opium derivatives, except for medical and scientific purposes. As a result, Britain rescheduled cannabis as a poison effective from April 1925. Thankfully it didn't last.

―――― HEROES OF HEMP: WILLIE NELSON ――――

COUNTRY AND WESTERN singer, Willie Nelson is the co-chair of the National Organization for the Reform of Marijuana Laws (NORML) and has sat on its advisory board for over a decade, fighting for marijuana legalization. In 2005 he hosted the first annual Willie Nelson & NORML Benefit Golf Tournament, which led to an appearance on the cover of the January 2008 issue of *High Times* magazine.

When Nelson's lung collapsed while swimming in 1981, and after suffering several bouts of pneumonia, he decided to quit either marijuana or tobacco—he chose the latter. In 2008 he started using a vaporizer to ease the strain on his lungs.

He has been arrested several times for possession of marijuana. The first was in 1974 in Dallas, Texas, then 20 years later in 1994, he was busted for a single marijuana cigarette in his car near Waco, Texas. On his way to a funeral in 2006, Nelson was busted yet again—this time in Louisiana—and charged with possession of marijuana and hallucinogenic mushrooms. He received six months probation. On November 26, 2010, Nelson was arrested in Sierra Blanca, Texas, for possession of six ounces of marijuana found in his tour bus. He was released on a $2,500 bail. After this last arrest he set up the TeaPot party.

In his 2012 autobiographical musings, *Roll Me Up and Smoke Me*

When I Die, the 80-year-old Nelson explained, "I thought, 'Hey there's a Tea Party, so why not a TeaPot Party?' There are now TeaPot Party representatives in every state of the union, and even in several foreign countries. On a few occasions, the TeaPot Party has backed a few politicians who believe, as we do, that marijuana should be legalized, taxed and regulated."

—— THE EMPEROR WEARS NO CLOTHES ——

POSSIBLY THE MOST IMPORTANT BOOK to be written about cannabis in the 20th century is Jack Herer's *The Emperor Wears No Clothes*. Published in 1985, it was the first book to investigate the real reasons why such a profitable and prodigious crop such as hemp was outlawed around the world. Herer was a late convert to cannabis, but became an ardent campaigner for its legalization, establishing Help End Marijuana Prohibition (HEMP). The book explores how hemp has been systematically erased from the collective consciousness as an indispensable, cheap, and plentiful tool for making paper, rope, clothes, cattle feed, and even plastics.

While the late Herer is seen as a bit of a hero in the cannabis counterculture (there's an award-winning strain of weed named after him), there are some European crop experts, like Dr. Hayo M. G. van der Werf, who think some of his claims about hemp as a panacea for the world's problems were grossly exaggerated. Ironically, *The Emperor Wears No Clothes* may be just that. However, there is still an unclaimed $100,000 reward for anyone who can disprove his research.

———————— CANNABIS & CRIME ————————

One of its detractors' favorite refrains is that cannabis is a dangerous drug that leads to a life of crime. Naysayers warned that legalizing cannabis would open the US to a terrifying crimewave. Of course anyone who's actually tried it probably has an inkling of how unlikely it is that consuming weed leads to violence and antisocial behavior (unless sitting in your room watching stupid videos for hours counts as antisocial behavior). And guess what—the statistics agree!

Since the relaxation of restrictions, authorities have seen a sharp decline in violent crime in states bordering Mexico, where violent crime has decreased by an average of 13% according to a 2017 report. The reason seems to be a decreased demand for illegal product since the legalization of medical marijuana. Meanwhile, in Colorado or Washington D.C., where the drug was first legalized for recreational use, reports suggest that legalization has had minimal, if any, effect on the crime rate.

> "It really puzzles me to see marijuana connected with narcotics, dope, and all that crap…it's a thousand times better than whiskey. It's an assistant—a friend."
> LOUIS ARMSTRONG, *Musician (1901–1971)*

GEORGE AND CHARLOTTE GO TO WHITE CASTLE

HOWEVER YOU FEEL ABOUT IT ethically and morally, it's standard scientific procedure to test new (and old) drugs on animals before progressing to human trials. The average citizen is far more enlightened about the unethical exploitation of animals now more than ever before—if only because of the plethora of real-time information we find ourselves bombarded with on a daily basis—so there are certain methods of research that we just won't countenance from the scientific community anymore. Despite this, scientists are still getting up to some strange shenanigans; here are a couple that involve marijuana, and not necessarily for the betterment of humankind:

In 1995, NASA thought it'd be a great idea to get spiders high on a variety of drugs and then see what kind of webs they wove. It *was* a great idea, and predictably the pothead spider gave up weaving his web about halfway through to wander off in search of Pringles. (Conversely, the LSD webs showed remarkable precision and intricacy.)

In 1974, the Heath/Tulane study set out to prove the adage that marijuana use kills brain cells. The study indicated that its test subjects, rhesus monkeys, were forced to inhale the equivalent of 30 joints a day; after 90 days they died and were found to have severe and permanent brain damage. It wasn't revealed until much later that the monkeys were actually administered daily doses of the equivalent of 63 joints through gas masks *in five minutes*. This means that every day the monkeys were deprived of oxygen for a full five minutes and the brain damage they suffered was due to suffocation, not marijuana. To this day there is no evidence that weed causes brain damage, permanent or otherwise.

HEROES OF HEMP: SOMA

THIS DREADLOCKED US-born herbal horticulturist started growing marijuana back in 1971. In 1996 he moved to Amsterdam where he set up his renowned Soma Seeds company, offering his award-winning seeds in the post to aspiring growers. He specializes in growing organic grass and medical marijuana, particularly after having open-heart surgery in 2005, and self-medicates with his own crops, prescribing 10–15 grams a day. He has won both the Cannabis Cup and the IC Growers cup three times, and 2007's Spannabis Champions Cup, and lectures as a "Ganja Guru" while regularly contributing to many magazines.

TOP TEN POT FICTION

Marihuana BY WILLIAM IRISH
(*Dell, 1941*)

Reefer Boy BY HAL ELLSON
(*Pedigree, 1957*)

The Marijuana Mob BY JAMES
HADLEY CHASE (*Eton, 1952*)

Marijuana Girl BY N. R.
DEMEXICO (*Beacon, 1960*)

Reefer Girl BY JANE MANNING
(*Cameo, 1953*)

Marijuana Murder BY
ANONYMOUS (*Superior, 1946*)

It Ain't Hay BY DAVID DODGE
(*Dell, 1946*)

Sex, Pot and Acid BY GEORGE
BAILEY (*Viceroy, 1968*)

Reefer Club BY LUKE ROBERTS
(*Stallion, 1953*)

Dope, Inc. BY JOACHIM JOESTEN
(*Avon, 1953*)

VENDING MACHINES

WE'RE AWARE THAT JUST THE concept of vending machines that dispense marijuana sounds like something only possible in a fantasyland where rainbows only have endings and unicorns roam freely across fields growing Twizzlers instead of grass, but this is serious. They exist.

With these vending machines already in use in medical dispensaries in the US, courtesy of California-based company Medbox Inc., other businesses are hoping to get in on the game and capitalize on weed's legality in Colorado and Washington. This probably doesn't mean we'll be seeing weed machines in every mall in America anytime soon, but it's very possible that a few years down the line, weed stores where the drug is legal will offer the automated option alongside the personal sales touch, and customers can choose according to their preference (and just for future reference, vending machines have already been designed to sell edible pot treats as well as pure bud).

COMEDY CANNABIS SONGS

BY THE GIGGLES IT INDUCES, it's no wonder there are plenty of funny marijuana tracks. Here's three of the best:

Soap Bar by **Goldie Lookin' Chain** (*Straight Outta Newport*, 2004)
The Welsh rappers spat lyrics extolling the joys of smoking cheap-ass hashish with this number: "Soap Bar's cheap, and so's my clothes, They've got to be cause of all the fucking holes, It tastes like shit and it makes you cough, And it's the fucking rubber in it that gets you off."

The Reefer Song by **Mindless Drug Hoover** (*Top Banana*, 1997)
This bizarre folky acoustic little ditty tells the tale of a cyclist who gets arrested and then proceeds to get the entire police station wasted: "Well I sold them two ounces and one 16th, and they rolled the biggest joint the world had ever seen…" Terribly remixed by The Orb.

Because I Got High by **Afroman** (*Because I Got High*, 2000)
Despite being a humorous track about a man whose entire life is destroyed by smoking dope, this song became a huge hit, reaching No. 1 in nine countries. It was the theme tune for Kevin Smith's film *Jay & Silent Bob Strike Back* (2001), and he went on to direct the music video.

WEST SIDE WEED

THE 1957 SONG *Gee, Officer Krupke*, from one of the best-loved musicals, *West Side Story*, had some very controversial cannabis-related lyrics by Stephen Sondheim:

Dear kindly Judge, your Honor,
My parents treat me rough.
With all their marijuana,
They won't give me a puff.

My father is a bastard,
My ma's an S.O.B.
My grandpa's always plastered,
My grandma pushes tea.

These original stage lyrics were changed slightly for the film version, but nevertheless kept the subtle nods to marijuana and "tea," which then later caused it to be banned by the BBC in 1962 because of the scandalous drug references. Years later, Sondheim stated he originally wanted it to be the first Broadway show to use the words "fuck" and "shit" in its song lyrics, with the end of the song being "Gee, Officer Krupke, Fuck you!" but in the end, the producers succeeded in softening it to "Krup you!"

HEROES OF HEMP: MR. NICE

HOWARD MARKS AKA "Mr. Nice," who died in April 2016, was the world's most notorious ex-cannabis smuggler. In his prime he was smuggling 30 tons of weed into the USA hidden inside a fictional rock band's speakers.

After making various connections in the early seventies, the Oxford graduate was soon smuggling hashish from Afghanistan, Lebanon, and Pakistan into Germany, Ireland, and the UK. By 1972 he was making £50,000 on each shipment. Regarding his smuggling as a service he deliberately avoided hard drugs recalling, "A dealer is really just someone who buys more dope than he can smoke. And I have to say, I'm ashamed, I tried to smoke it all. There was just too fuckin' much of it."

As Marks recalled in his 1996 autobiography, *Mr. Nice*, "Between 1975 and 1978, 24 loads totaling 55,000 pounds of marijuana and hashish had been successfully imported through John F. Kennedy Airport, New York. They had involved the Mafia, the Yakuza, the Brotherhood of Eternal Love, the Thai army, the Palestine Liberation Organization, the Pakistani Armed Forces, Nepalese monks, and other individuals from all walks of life. The total profit made by all concerned was $48,000,000. They'd had a good run."

Incredibly, the Welshman made contacts with the IRA, MI6, and the CIA, with the latter even setting up a $300,000 cannabis deal with Marks. Unfortunately, it all went wrong when the contact died and US Customs seized the haul.

In 1988 he was eventually caught by the US Drug Enforcement Agency, extradited from Spain to the States, and was sentenced to 25 years in a maximum security prison, but released after seven in 1995.

By the end of his life, Marks had racked up an impressive CV as a writer, public speaker, activist, and occasional DJ. He was also a leading voice in the demand for the legalization of grass in the UK, and even stood for Parliament in the 1997 UK elections. His book was adapted into a 2010 film, also called *Mr. Nice*, and he was played by fellow Welshman, Rhys Ifans.

--------- MAKING HASH ---------

TAKING THE STICKY CANNABIS resin formed by the trichomes (glands) of the female plant, hashish can be made in one of three ways. Firstly, dried buds are sieved—either mechanically or by hand—through gauze and the residue powder is heat compressed into blocks. The second method involves filtering the buds with iced water. This allows the precious trichomes (which contain the active THC) to sink to the bottom while the leaves and stalks float. The residue is then filtered to purify it further, and is known as "bubble-hash." This is because you can test the purity of the hash by adding heat to it. The more it bubbles, the better the quality. The third method is to chemically extract the resin using solvents like ethanol, which is then evaporated, and forms a "honey oil" or "hash oil," but purists tend to avoid this method as the process breaks down the trichomes. The trouble with hash is that many unscrupulous dealers cut it with various adherents to stretch the product further. Notorious "Soap Bar" has been known to contain everything from plastics to engine oil, and even faeces. So just make sure your shit is good shit and not shit shit.

> "The illegality of cannabis is outrageous, an impediment to full utilization of a drug which helps produce the serenity and insight, sensitivity and fellowship so desperately needed in this increasingly mad and dangerous world."
>
> CARL SAGAN, *Astrophysicist (1934–1996)*

--------- 4:20 ---------

ALSO WRITTEN AS 420, this mysterious number has long been a secret code for tokers. Many theories have developed about its origins, from being the number of various legal acts and bills, or amount of active chemicals in cannabis, to even the date of Bob Marley's death (actually May 11th, 1981), but none of these are true. The real origin of these curious digits goes way back to the early seventies in San Rafael, California when a bunch of stoner students, known as "the Waldos," needed a code for arranging a smoking session. The number referred to the time, 4:20pm, so fellow stoners could pass in the corridors saying "420, [insert location]?" without fear of being busted. The phrase spread virally until in became common parlance, a decade later, for asking if someone had weed or to simply identify a fellow smoker. Nowadays it's associated with April 20th as an unofficial date to celebrate weed.

PICK YOUR HIGH

ALTHOUGH CANNABIS GROWS IN THREE main strains—sativa, indica, and ruderalis—herbal horticulturists have spent decades constantly mixing and matching genetic strains, looking for the perfect high, tailored to smokers' requirements. For example, Strawberry Cough has a fruity flavor to it, while Purple Kush produces a heavy and mellow high. These are seeded from either sativa, indica, or a blend of the two.

Breeding requires pollinating a female plant with male pollen. The males —identified by their ball-like stamen—are separated from female plants to prevent accidental fertilization and to allow more control over which male is used. The selected male pollen is then sprinkled on the female flowers. The resultant seeds have the characteristics of both plants. It's a tricky business as the seeds can often be infertile. If this is the case then crossbreeding needs to be stabilized by "cubing." This process involves finding specific traits in the new hybrid plant (such as increased resin production) that match traits in a stable parent plant and then breeding the two. This process sometimes needs to be repeated two or three times (hence the term cubing) before the strain is stable enough to breed by itself.

Today there are hundreds of strains to pick from, including Super Silver Haze, Northern Lights, Kryptonite, Champagne, Shiskaberry, Big Bud, White Widow, Western Winds, Kali Mist, G13, and endless Skunk varieties. The list continues to expand as farmers seek new ways to get people stoned.

HEROES OF HEMP: ROB VAN DAM

AMERICAN PROFESSIONAL wrestler Rob Van Dam has been a vocal proponent of the use and legalization of weed for the entirety of his 20-plus-year career. Even an arrest for 18 grams of marijuana in 2006 has not deterred him; if anything, it's made him more determined to fight for pot's cause.

In addition to occasionally contributing opinion pieces to *Cannabis Culture* magazine, he's incorporated the 4:20 aesthetic into his merchandize and was featured in *High Times* magazine in 1999.

When most high-profile wrestlers were hiding their habits in shame, afraid of the drug-using athlete stigma, Van Dam spoke out about the medicinal benefits, physical and mental, of cannabis, and even claimed that marijuana makes him a better athlete. In 2009 he spoke at the NORML National Conference, and he continues to advocate smoking in the media at every opportunity. For his tireless campaigning on behalf of this medicinal of herbs, Rob Van Dam takes his well-earned place among the exalted Heroes of Hemp.

ACRONYM: CDB

The second most active cannabinoid in marijuana, cannabidiol (CDB) is thought to act as a counterbalance to its more psychoactive cousin, THC. Its sedative effect means that potential medical uses include easing epilepsy, spasms, anxiety disorders, bipolar disorder, and schizophrenia. Research has even shown that it helps halt the growth of cancer cells.

> "I believe in individual rights. I mean, I would like
> to see everybody be able to smoke pot."
>
> SUSAN SARANDON, *Actress and Activist (b. 1946)*

KNOW YOUR STUFF: WHAT'S HYDROPONIC WEED?

"I GET HIGH ON HYDROPONIC WEED..." sang Lana del Rey in "Brooklyn Baby." But what the hell are hydroponics and why is everyone talking about them these days??

Hydroponic marijuana is simply marijuana that's been grown in a solution of water and nutrients instead of soil, meaning it's grown in a more controlled environment for quicker growth, greater yields, and a more uniform crop. You might hear that hydroponic weed is stronger than soil-grown marijuana, but it really depends on the strength of the particular strain that's been cultivated. Hydroponic weed may therefore have a higher THC content, but only because that's what people are choosing to grow, and the crop is more consistent.

DAMNED IF YOU DO, DAMNED IF YOU DON'T

ON THE RECREATIONAL DRUG scale of harm, marijuana is perceived to be at the lowest end, causing the fewest negative side effects while having a high positive value to the user. The drug's ability to calm is probably the most cited reason for use, so it's no surprise that many people with anything from daily stress to diagnosed anxiety disorders choose to self-medicate with weed. But for all its soporific qualities, marijuana can also cause anxiety and, in particular, panic attacks. In fact, anywhere from 20 to 30 percent of smokers report having panic attacks after smoking. The mechanics of weed's ability to cause anxiety isn't yet understood—it could be genetic or it could be that many smokers have anxiety problems to begin with—but it seems that first-timers are the most susceptible. Novices take note: always use the buddy system. Safety first.

> "Some people are just better high."
> JUSTIN TIMBERLAKE, *Musician (b. 1981)*

MARIJUANA AS A (POTENTIAL) CHEMICAL WEAPON

IN THE 1960S, US ARMY Colonel Dr. James Ketchum conducted experiments involving marijuana and mind control at the Edgewood Arsenal in Maryland. Edgewood was the headquarters of the US Army Chemical Corps, and Chief of Clinical Research Ketchum intended to build a new kind of chemical weapon, one that would incapacitate the enemy without immediate damage or long-term harm—most likely by sending them to sleep for an extended period or inducing almost paralyzing attacks of the giggles. Ketchum dreamed of a "war without death," and used a highly potent, synthetic form of marijuana to try to achieve it.

The subjects of the Army experiments were soldiers who volunteered, and the trials were conducted under rigorously controlled scientific conditions. One potent THC compound and one stereoisomer produced satisfying effects: the compound caused a volunteer to find everything funny and have trouble raising his arms, and the stereoisomer effected a significant drop in blood pressure, causing the subjects to faint and have trouble moving. Unfortunately, in Ketchum's opinion, the Army decided a sudden drop in blood pressure could be dangerous and suspended trials, thereby eliminating the possibility of a non-lethal, marijuana-based chemical weapon.

HOW DO YOU TAKE YOURS?

SMOKING IT IN A JOINT MAY BE THE CLASSIC WAY to take cannabis, but if you're taking it for medical reasons, you might not want your hit combusted. Here's a helpful roundup of alternative ways to consume the heavenly herb—and what you effects you can expect from them...

Eat: Make a batch of cannabutter (see page 73) and the culinary world is your oyster, so to speak. You can cook up a cannabis feast with anything that requires a good slab of butter; alternatively, you can use an oil concentrate. Expect the effects to kick in after a couple of hours, and be prepared for a much more intense high than you get when smoking.

Drink: Chemical compounds can be extracted in an alcoholic tincture (see below)—which makes for some fun party drinks, or a low-calorie alternative to hash brownies. Tinctures make it easier to control the dose, but, as with eating, the effects will be delayed so remember to pace yourself.

Tincture: An alcohol-based cannabis infusion that can be applied in drops under the tongue or added to food and drink. When taken directly, it enters the bloodstream immediately, which allows for good dose control. Just make sure you don't overdo it on the first go!

Smoke: Smoking from a joint or bong can be a sociable activity; a little bit of weed or hash in a pipe gives you a quick one-hit wonder. Effects will be felt immediately, though vary according to your method, strength of the strain, and amount you consume. Remember to breathe between hits.

Vaporize: A similar method of consumption to smoking, vaporizers gently heat the cannabis to release its chemical compounds, giving you a cleaner, better-tasting high. Vaporizers come in different forms, including hand-held and table-top devices.

Dab: This method involves inhaling a dose of cannabis concentrate from a heated surface like a nail. It's a fast-acting and extremely potent method (if the oil is high in THC) so caution is advised, and best avoided altogether if you're new to cannabis consumption.

Rub: Cannabis lotions and balms, called topicals, can be applied directly to the skin for high-less, localized pain-relief.

——— HOLY COW HOT CHOCOLATE ———

THIS IS SIMPLY DELICIOUS, even without the holy herb added.

1 cup/250ml milk
5 tbsp granulated sugar
1 cup/250ml single cream
pinch of ground cinnamon
½ tsp vanilla extract

⅛oz/4g cannabis finely ground
5oz/150g plain chocolate
1 small chocolate bar,
whipped cream and/or baby
marshmallows to decorate

Instructions:

1 Gently heat the milk and sugar in a pan until the sugar dissolves.
Then add all the other ingredients, apart from the chocolate and other
toppings.

2 Bring to the boil, then simmer for abut one hour. Then pour the resulting
"cannamilk" through a coffee filter.

3 Put the cannamilk back in the pan, break up the chocolate, drop
it in, and gently heat until melted, stirring all the time.

4 Pour into a mug and decorate with whipped cream, marshmallows
and grated chocolate. Yum!

EIGHT THINGS TO DO
WHEN YOU'RE STONED

AS EVERYBODY KNOWS, almost everything is better when you're high, but these eight things were made for weed:

Get out in nature: Even if it's just the park. Watch the sun rise, stare at leaves rustling on trees, find shapes in clouds, and find kinship with the beasts. Smoking weed outside is awesome.

Listen to music: Best done at a festival, but effective even in your bedroom. Great for discovering new music, but you might come back to a band a while later and wonder what it was you saw in their music—in which case, just get high again.

Eat food: The best thing I've ever tasted was fish goujons ordered after a great session in the park. Salty or sweet food is best. For bonus points combine eating delicious food with getting high (see our brownie recipe on page 15).

Write down your ideas: You will probably have great ideas while stoned—great ideas for bands, great ideas for songs, great ideas about fixing the world's problems...—but you need to make sure you write them down, otherwise you might forget them.

Watch a movie: Everything is funnier when you're high, so make the most of it and watch a classic stoner flick (see page 8). If you're feeling more epic than giggly, try a nature documentary and prepare to say "AWWWWWWSOME" quite a lot!

Clean your house: Seriously? Yes seriously. When you're high, mindless, repetitive activities can become really, really absorbing. Proof, no, that weed solves most things!

Make Art: Just like you have great ideas when stoned, you'll also be capable of more original and interesting artworks. Top tip: get your materials ready and start scribbling before you spark up.

Make love: Oh yes, yes, yes! And finally: for more intense lovemaking, just add the holy herb...

RELIGION

DESPITE PREDOMINANTLY being associated with Rastafarianism and Coptics, many religions have used marijuana in rituals. Japanese Shintoism celebrates hemp as a symbol of purity, with offerings of the plant (along with rice and salt) made to the divine Kami. Shinto priests wave a gohei wand made of hemp fibers over worshippers dressed in hemp paper robes in an act of cleansing. Small government-sanctioned plantations also exist where the hemp is grown to supply temples with sacred rope and other materials for these rituals. The Middle Eastern Sufis also regard cannabis, or kaif, as sacred and use it in a similar way as Rastafarians—as a means of communicating or getting closer to Allah. Other religions connected to the use of marijuana include Tantric Buddhism, Hinduism, and ancient Pagan rituals.

SKUNK

THE MOST NOTORIOUS STRAIN of weed, Skunk has a strong, heady aroma, hence the name. Mostly grown hydroponically, the Sativa-dominant weed has a much higher THC level (10–15 percent) than other strains and very little CBD. This is great for getting that instant head rush and a very strong high, but the lack of the CBD has caused some concerns for heavy smokers. Some scientists believe that ingesting high levels of THC encourages schizophrenia and other mental disorders. There are at least 11 different sub-strains of Skunk, including Cheese, Amnesia, and the slightly ominous-sounding Deathskünk.

——— COMPLETE LIST OF WINNERS: ———
THE AMSTERDAM CANNABIS CUP 1988-2014

1988—SKUNK #1
by Cultivator's Choice

1989—EARLY PEARL/SKUNK #1
X NORTHERN LIGHTS #5/HAZE
by the Seed Bank, Snocap by David Swenson

1990—NORTHERN LIGHTS #5
by the Seed Bank

1991—SKUNK BALLS *by Free City*

1992—HAZE X SKUNK #1
by Homegrown Fantasy

1993—HAZE X NORTHERN
LIGHTS #5
by Sensi Seed Bank

1994—JACK HERER
by Sensi Seed Bank

1995—WHITE WIDOW
by Green House

1996—WHITE RUSSIAN
by De Dampkring

1997—PEACE MAKER
by De Dampkring

1998—SUPER SILVER HAZE
by Green House

1999—SUPER SILVER HAZE
by Green House

2000—BLUEBERRY *by the Noon*

2001—SWEET TOOTH *by Barney's*

2002—MORNING GLORY
by Barney's

2003—HAWAIIAN SNOW
by Green House

2004—AMNESIA HAZE
by Barney's

2005—WILLIE NELSON
by Barney's

2006—ARJAN'S ULTRA HAZE #1
by Green House

2007—G-13 HAZE
by Barney's

2008—SUPER LEMON HAZE
by Green House

2009—SUPER LEMON HAZE
by Green House

2010—TANGERINE DREAM
by Barney's

2011—LIBERTY HAZE
by Barney's

2012—FLOWER BOMB KUSH
by Green House

2013—ROLLEX OG KUSH
by Green Place

2014—COOKIES KUSH
by Barney's

HEROES OF HEMP: KEVIN SMITH

K EVIN SMITH HAS NEVER SHIED away from speaking about his special relationship with marijuana. He claims he didn't become a "hard-core stoner" until after *Zack and Miri Make a Porno* bombed at the box office (2008)—apparently he was introduced to pot in a serious way by Seth Rogen—and some critics mark that moment as the beginning of the end of his filmmaking career. However, Jay and Silent Bob were dealers in *Clerks* (1994), Smith's fictional comic-book characters Bluntman and Chronic appeared in *Chasing Amy* back in 1997 and became an actual comic book written by Smith in 2001, and his comic store in New Jersey is called Jay and Silent Bob's Secret Stash, which could be a euphemism for…something. Whatever his actual history with the drug, Smith has stated publicly that heavy smoking has focused his work ethic and actually increased his creative output, which goes some way to dispelling the slacker myth. Maybe.

TEN CLASSIC GRASS STRAINS

(By strength)

1 JACK HERER *****	**6** SILVER HAZE****
2 SAGE****	**7** WHITE RUSSIAN***
3 WHITE WIDOW****	**8** AK-47***
4 YUMBOLDT****	**9** BUBBLEGUM***
5 WARLOCK HAZE****	**10** K2**

PAPERS

THE MOST POPULAR way of smoking marijuana is by rolling a joint, for which you need good rolling papers, or skins. In the bad old days this would involve gluing together small papers (3" or 78mm long) to make a doobie worth smoking, but eventually manufacturers caught on and started making king-size versions, around 4" (100mm) long, which made skinning up that much easier. These days there's an endless variety to choose from, including flavored (liquorice, grape, and banana), rolls (such as Rips) that allow enormous joints to be created, pre-rolled cones that you just fill with gear, and even honey-dipped tobacco leaves for rolling blunts. Of course, aficionados use only hemp paper to roll their own.

HARRY J. ANSLINGER

I F THE STORY OF MARIJUANA has a single villain it's Harry J. Anslinger. An ardent anti-drug campaigner ever since he heard the screams of a morphine addict at the age of 12, Anslinger was made Assistant Prohibition Commissioner in the Bureau of Prohibition. Promoted to Commissioner of the Federal Bureau of Narcotics in 1930, he was alarmed by the growing use of cannabis as a possible replacement for opiate abuse, and made it his mission to make marijuana illegal. It was already restricted in several states, but Anslinger set about with a zeal to have it banned on a Federal level.

He teamed up with William Randolph Hearst's newspapers, creating a scare campaign, using cases like Victor Licata, who axed his family to death—supposedly under the influence of marijuana. He warned, "Marihuana is a shortcut to the insane asylum. Smoke marihuana cigarettes for a month and what was once your brain will be nothing but a storehouse of horrid specters. Hasheesh makes a murderer who kills for the love of killing out of the mildest mannered man who ever laughed at the idea that any habit could ever get him…" He ran radio campaigns and even supported the making of Dwain Esper's sensational 1935 cannabis exposé, *Assassin of Youth.*

He was also a blatant racist, using his discrimination as a reason for pot prohibition, "Colored students at the Univ. of Minn. partying with (white) female students, smoking [marijuana] and getting their sympathy with stories of racial persecution. Result: pregnancy…" He actively targeted jazz musicians in his campaign, seeing several arrested for possession, including Gene Krupa and Louis Armstrong.

Eventually, in 1937, Anslinger's hate campaign against hemp succeeded with the passing of the Marijuana Tax Act, which effectively outlawed cannabis in America. Not resting on his laurels, he also managed to convince other countries to join the ongoing prohibition. Having spent 32 years railing against weed, he finally retired in 1962 and passed on to the Great Bureau in the Sky on November, 14, 1975. His vilifying policies did more harm to the harmless stoner than any other politician or government body before or since.

> "I went to Vietnam, and I was there for a long time…
> [Using marijuana] made the difference between staying human or,
> as Michael Douglas said, becoming a beast. I'm telling you, it's rough
> and a lot of people in that platoon used it, not on the front line
> but in the back, to stay in touch with themselves."
>
> OLIVER STONE, *Director (b. 1946)*

THE FABULOUS FURRY FREAK BROTHERS

THE PERENNIAL STONER TRIO of Phineas, Freewheelin' Franklin, and Fat Freddy (and not forgetting the latter's cat), first appeared in 1968 when creator Gilbert Shelton drew them for the Texan underground paper, *The Rag*. Inspired by the Marx Brothers and the Three Stooges, Shelton printed 3,000 copies of the first comic and sold a few hundred in Austin before heading to San Francisco, the then home of underground comix, to sell the rest and set up Rip Off Press publishing company.

Initially, the strips were just about everyday pothead concerns, like getting high, getting laid, claiming welfare, and trying to avoid being arrested by narks (narcotics officers). But Shelton, assisted by Paul Mavrides and Dave Sheridan, started more ambitious storylines creating multi-part, globe-spanning epics like *Grass Roots*, where the boys find a "year's supply" of cocaine and move to the country with the proceeds, and *The Idiots Abroad*.

There have been numerous attempts at transferring the tokin' trio to the big screen, either as live action or, most recently in 2008, as claymation. But as yet none has been successful. Knockabout, The Freak Bros.' UK publisher since the late seventies, released an Omnibus in 2008 that collected every single trippy strip to date, even the rare color one that appeared in *Playboy*.

The 14 comics have remained almost continuously in print for over 40 years, with the three unrelated "brothers" still entertaining thousands of stoners with every new generation that discover them. There is an unfinished Freak Brothers story set on a houseboat in Amsterdam with the aged trio, and Shelton has said, "…Perhaps one of these days we'll get back on that project, especially if we can find a way to hire a couple of dozen more artists." But with it being over 100 pages, and Shelton's increasing age, it's looking unlikely.

---

10 CLASSIC HASHISH TYPES

(By strength)

1 NEPALESE TEMPLE BALLS*****	**6** WHITE WIDOW****
2 MELANA CREAM*****	**7** SUPER KETMA****
3 ROYAL NEPALESE*****	**8** AFGHANI BLACK****
4 JELLYHASH*****	**9** GOLD LEBANESE***
5 NORTHERN LIGHTS****	**10** SHEEBA***

A MYSTERY EVEN MYSTERY, INC. COULDN'T SOLVE

TECHNICALLY, THEY'RE THE ONLY ONES who *could* solve it, but they're not talking. Children's TV of the 70s and 80s ran the gambit from subversive to outright trippy, but the most overt alleged allusion to marijuana use has to be Norville Rogers—better known as "Shaggy"—from the cartoon *Scooby Doo*. He, along with his constant companion Scooby, just had that vibe of the habitual smoker about him. But those involved with the show—including radio legend Casey Kasem, who voiced Shaggy for twenty-five years—maintained he was just a goofy product of the times. Fans have always wondered, though, especially after they grew up and were able to make more informed connections. On the one hand, Shaggy's portrayed as your garden-variety hippie slacker—long haired, shabbily dressed (bell bottoms!), and a bit slow on the uptake. On the other hand . . . well, let's look at the evidence, shall we?

Exhibit A: Shaggy is from a town called Coolsville. Literally, that is actually the town he's from. This may or may not have anything to do with him being an alleged smoker, but it needs to be said. *Coolsville.*

Exhibit B: "A bit slow on the uptake" could equate to a bit stoned. Shaggy often seems to have no idea where he was or how he got there, a little surprised about what was going on but on the whole okay with it. In other words, he's high.

Exhibit C: Shaggy and Scooby clearly live in the back of a van. A Mystery Machine, no less. It's like a magic carpet ride but smoother and a little low-rent.

Exhibit D: Shaggy and Scooby constantly have the munchies. They are shoving food in their faces 24/7 like Doritos are going out of style. What's that about weed increasing appetite?

Exhibit E: Shaggy says "like," like, all the time. Because that's what happens, like, when people's brains are moving at, like, one-fifth of their normal, like, speed and they need to punctuate the, like, silence to make it sound like they're still, like, paying attention.

Exhibit F: Um . . . what were we talking about?

There will probably never be a clear answer to whether Shaggy was a stoner, because he was and is, after all, the star of a children's show. But to be honest, we'd all be a bit disappointed if any of the creators came out and said he was, because it's much for fun to have our own mystery to solve. And we would solve it, too, if it weren't for those meddling kids!

ALL THAT JAZZ

LONG BEFORE REGGAE AND RAPPERS became associated musical champions of wacky baccy there was another group of performers who were inspired by the marijuana muse: jazz musicians. Known as "tea" in the twenties, thirties, and forties, grass was inspiring Cab Calloway to sing about "that funny reefer man" in 1932. Another jazz term for a stoner or grass was a viper, and in 1938 Sidney Bechet & Noble Sissles Swinster's sang "I'm viper mad."

Between 1943–1950 The Narcotics Bureau attacked the jazz scene and lots of musicians were arrested in the crackdown, including drummer Gene Kruper—who received a three-month jail sentence for just two joints—and Louis Armstrong, who was lucky enough to get off with a suspended sentence. Armstrong was a vocal proponent of the herb even recording his 1928 paean to it, *Muggles* (slang for marijuana) and he wrote in his memoirs, "It really puzzles me to see marijuana connected with narcotics…dope and all that crap. It's a thousand times better than whiskey—it's an assistant—a friend."

But the king of them all was Milton "Mezz" Mezzrow. The clarinetist/saxophonist was arrested in 1940 for possession of 60 joints entering a jazz club, with intent to supply. He became such a renowned dealer to fellow musicians that his name became synonymous with marijuana, and he was immortalized in Stuff Smith and the Onyx Boys' classic, *You'se a Viper*: "Dreamed about a reefer, Five foot long, The mighty Mezz, but not too strong, You'll be high, but for long, Cuz you'se a viper…"

MARIJUANA TINCTURE

WHILE THE THC IN MARIJUANA can be broken down in fats and oils, it can also be extracted in alcohol, and consequently powerful cocktails await those who are prepared to put the effort into making a tincture. Here's how.

You'll need:

3–4oz/22g Marijuana leaves and/or buds

3floz/90ml of 40–70% proof alcohol

Something sweet, like a peach schnapps or a brandy, is better

than vodka, to hide the bitterness

Muslin or a coffee filter

Funnel

Dark green, blue or brown glass bottle with an airtight screw lid

Instructions:

1 Grind up the marijuana into a fine powder and soak overnight in warm water. This removes any water-soluble impurities while leaving in the THC.

2 The following morning, drain off the water using the muslin/coffee filter and scoop the damp powder into the glass bottle and pour the alcohol on top.

3 Give it a good shake and store the bottle in a cool, dark place for ten days, and shake daily. After ten days it's ready to use, but the longer you leave it, the stronger it gets.

4 Then filter the grass out with the muslin/coffee filter, keeping the liquid and discarding the now inert grass. You can repeat steps 1–3 again with fresh cannabis to increase the potency, but I wouldn't!

5 You can drink the tincture straight or add it to a cocktail, or use in cooking.

MAHJOUN

IN THE 11TH CENTURY, Middle Eastern Arabs were prevented by Islam from drinking alcohol. However, they were allowed to consume cannabis, so they took lumps of hashish, dried fruit, nuts, and honey, and pulverized it into a sweet sticky treat known as mahjoun. The recipe spread all over the Arabic world, including Morocco, where it was sometimes made with alternative ingredients of small doses of the narcotic plants datura and belladonna, and butter and gum Arabic.

THE MUNCHIES: SCIENCE OR PSYCHOLOGY?

THERE IS AN OVERWHELMING AMOUNT of anecdotal evidence suggesting that marijuana use increases appetite, so much so that the phenomenon has been given a name all of its own: "the munchies." While it's been theorized that the munchies is a psychological side-effect of smoking—the drug lowers inhibitions and gluttony is often at the top of the vice list—there is in fact a physiological basis for the marriage of marijuana and Taco Bell.

It was previously believed that marijuana, like all drugs, acted primarily on the brain and so if the munchies were in fact a physical response to smoking, it would be because it changed the perception of how food tastes by bonding to the appropriate brain receptors. But a recent study by the Monell Chemical Senses Center in Philadelphia, Pennsylvania, and Kyushu University in Japan has found that the cannabinoids in weed—which ape the naturally occurring, appetite-inducing endocannabinoids in the body—directly affect the taste buds, making foods seem sweeter to the smoker.

The Monell Center believes that this breakthrough in roach research could pave the way to new methods of treating obesity, diabetes, and lost appetite as a result of other diseases. If you needed yet another argument for the legalization of medical marijuana, you're welcome. Pay it forward by writing to your local government representative or moving to California.

THE CANNABIS CUP

GROWING WEED is its own reward, but serious herbal horticulturists can enter their prized plants to compete for a cup in various festivals around the world. Back in the day there was only one event that really counted: The Cannabis Cup in Amsterdam. Launched in 1988 by activist and High Times editor, Steve Hager the show allowed anyone to pay to become a judge, with the highest number reaching 2,300 in 2008. 2012's winner was Flower Bomb Kush, an incredibly fast-growing strain that flowers in five-and-a-half weeks instead of the average eight, and was described by one of the judges as "strong Kush taste similar to Purple Kush and nice couch lock high…that shit was booooom!" The Amsterdam chapter was closed in 2014 after authorities threatened to shut down the expo and arrest all participants on the morning the show was due to begin. Fortunately, the event had already crossed the ocean, and April 2013 saw the first US iteration of The Cannabis Cup take place in Denver, Colorado, with 15,000 people turning up. There are now events throughout the year all across the country.

HOW TO ROLL A JOINT

THERE'S A MILLION DIFFERENT WAYS to skin-up and as always creativity rules. For the novice you'll need some cigarettes, a lighter, some king-size rolling papers, some thin cardboard and, of course, some hash or grass!

1 If mixing with tobacco (advisable for newbies) run a flame down a cigarette to dry the tobacco out. Then lick your finger and run it down the length of the cigarette and tear the moist strip off allowing the contents to drop onto the king-size paper. Alternatively, simply hold the cigarette upside down and gently roll it between your fingers and let the tobacco sprinkle out over the paper.

2 Tear off a thin strip of cardboard and roll it up tightly and place at one end of the paper. This is the "roach." You can buy pads of ready-to-roll roach paper, or the more health conscious may want to use a filter instead.

3 Grind up your grass as small as possible so that it burns evenly, or heat the hash with a lighter so that it crumbles easily, and then sprinkle along the length of the joint.

4 Gently pick up the paper and roll it between your forefingers and thumb, taking care not to drop the contents on the floor.

5 Carefully lick the gummed strip of the paper—make sure it's not too wet (no one likes a soggy joint and it won't light)—and roll over and seal it. Don't pack it too tight, as air needs to flow through.

6 Twist the end, light, and enjoy!

Note: *This can take years of practice to get it just right!*

RASTAFARIANISM

THE "SACRED 'ERB" or ganja, is a central tenant of the Rastafarian religion, and Rastafarians believe that smoking weed purifies the body and mind, bringing them closer to Jah (God). Using the Bible as the justification for toking, they quote many passages including: *Genesis 1:29* "And God said, Behold, I have given you every herb-bearing seed, which is upon the face of all the earth, and every tree, is the fruit of a tree yielding seed; to you it shall be for meat;" *Genesis 3:18* "...thou shalt eat the herb of the field;" and *Psalms 104:14* "He causeth the grass to grow for the cattle, and herb for the service of man," among others. As they point out, weed is a gift from God.

Rastas use ganja (from the Sanskrit, *ganjika*) in two main ways. Reasoning involves one honored member lighting up and passing the sacrament round while matters of Jah are discussed. The joint, or chalice, is passed clockwise, except in times of war when it's passed in the opposite direction. The other time grass is taken is on holy days known as Groundation or Binghi, such as July, 23—their spiritual leader, Haile Selassie's birthday. These are marked by days of singing, feasting, dancing, and smoking.

The use of marijuana has caused much conflict for Rastas over the years, seeing them persecuted across the globe. In 1998 Janet Reno, the US Attorney General, said that Rastafarians did not have the religious right to smoke grass, and in the UK this ban apparently does not contravene the European Convention on Human Rights. However, the more progressive Italian Supreme Court changed their laws in 2008, allowing Rastafarians larger possessions of ganja for sacrament.

"I've been smoking weed for forty-four years, five nights a week...
I'm the poster boy to prove it doesn't do you much harm."
LEE CHILD, *Writer (b. 1954)*

— AFTER-SCHOOL SPECIAL: JUST SAY NO! —

ALMOST EVERY AMERICAN WHO WAS a tween or teen between the early seventies and late nineties will be well-versed in the After School Special oeuvre, but here's a little run-down to get the younger—or older—kids up to date. Over 25 years, ABC produced a series of melodramatic made-for-TV movies aimed at educating the youth about the dangers of being young. Topics given the teen treatment included divorce, death, illiteracy, peer pressure, and, of course, drugs.

Stoned, broadcast in 1980 and starring heartthrob-to-be Scott Baio, starts off as a primer in how to smoke, with good-boy Baio choking on some joint smoke and then graduating quickly to a bong (mostly unlit). He quickly gains friends, confidence, giggles, and game, but loses interest in school. He's warned that "marywana" causes chromosome damage, birth defects, and sterility (according to a "government survey"), but Baio just doesn't take the hype seriously, and continues on his path of self-destruction. After he almost kills his brother in a rowboat accident due to grass-induced negligence (but ends up only destroying his hopes and dreams instead), Baio sees the error of his ways and sets the bong aside.

Stoned takes a different tack than the usual gateway drug malarkey fed to children of a certain era, in that it focuses on the dangers of using drugs to escape adolescent problems. But the real moral here is clear: friends don't let friends row stoned.

—————— SMUGGLING'S A NO-NO ——————

EVER THOUGHT ABOUT "DOING A HOWARD MARKS" and smuggling harmless weed around the world? Here's a list of countries you should *definitely avoid* trafficking in, as they all carry the death penalty. Some countries like China and Singapore are avid executioners, whereas others, like the Philippines, repealed the death sentence in 2006.

Saudi Arabia	China
Malaysia	United Arab Emirates
Indonesia	Thailand
Singapore	Egypt

Technically, the USA reserves the right to execute anyone trafficking over 60,000 kilos, or 60,000 plants, but thankfully this law has never been enforced. In June 2013, British pensioner, Charles Ferndale, was sentenced to be hanged for smuggling in three tons of cannabis (worth \$4.6/£2.9 million) into Egypt from Pakistan, along with four others. You have been warned!

SOUTH AFRICA

I N SOUTH AFRICA CANNABIS is known as "Dagga," and it grows from the border of Mozambique, in the North, all the way down the Eastern Cape to Port Elizabeth. South Africa preempted America's prohibition of grass by banning it in 1928, but regardless, this "Green Gold" is the main source of income for thousands of people. Today, Dagga is sold in various ways from wraps, called "fingers," bags known as "bankies," in matchboxes, and tied up in "Malawi cobs" (similar to Thai sticks), and it's incredibly cheap by US standards. A whole kilo can cost as little as 90 rand (£6 or US$10).

Local strains like the legendary Durban Poison (with its uplifting cerebral high), Malawi Gold, and Swazi Red are held in high regard by connoisseurs. But it's important not to get Dagga confused with Wild Dagga, a completely different plant, *Leonotis leonurus*, or Lion's Tail. Funnily enough this other Dagga is part of the mint family, but can also be used like cannabis, but has a weaker high, and is occasionally used as a substitute. While technically legal in the US, the smoke is supposedly unpleasant and rough, so many use the dried leaves in a minty tea. The main psychoactive component of *Leonotis leonurus* is leonurine, which acts in a similar way to THC in marijuana.

THE REAL COSTS OF AMERICA'S "WAR ON DRUGS"

I N 2010 over 656,000 Americans were arrested on marijuana charges, and on average, an American is arrested for violating cannabis laws every 30 seconds. More money is spent on law enforcement than on prevention and treatment combined. And fighting the war on drugs isn't cheap either. It costs the state of Florida $1.9 billion a year to prosecute offenders and a staggering $3 billion in New York. In 2013 the Cato Institute estimated that the US Government could save $13.7 billion a year if marijuana wasn't prohibited.

ETYMOLOGY: SINSEMILLA (NOUN)

Circa 1975, from the Mexican Spanish, *sin semilla*, literally meaning "without seed." The technique of growing cannabis where only the unpollinated female plant is allowed to blossom, without seeds being formed, thus giving large panicled flowers ("buds") that have a high content of cannabinoids.

THE SLACKER MYTH

FOR YEARS POT SMOKING has been stigmatized by "the slacker myth"—apart from all the cancers, infertility, and brain damage we've been warned about, it's been said that pot also makes you stupid, forgetful, and lazy. Stoner representation in movies has been squarely set in the "loser" camp for decades, even in films that aren't necessarily anti-marijuana. Think Jeff Spicoli in *Fast Times at Ridgemont High* (1982), Travis in *Clueless* (1995), The Dude in *The Big Lebowski* (1998), Brian in *Half Baked* (1998), and Cheech & Chong among many, many others. We're not saying they're not heroes in their own right, but these characters are usually jobless, feckless, and muddling through life limited by a cocoon of smoke.

Outside of fiction, however, some of our most productive young people are crediting marijuana for their success, at least in part. Seth Rogen smokes while he writes, and his output has been vast and of quality; pro-wrestler Rob Van Dam has won 21 championships, mostly while high; author Alexandre Dumas loved his hash; Bob Marley did all right for himself; Sir Richard Branson, he of the vast business empire, is a fan; travel guru Rick Steves is a member of the National Organization for the Reform of Marijuana Laws and credits pot with making him a better travel writer...The list of successful potheads is just too long to enumerate here.

Times are changing and with a younger generation of successful professionals speaking out about their productive relationships with cannabis, the slacker stereotype is sure to crumble. Eventually.

WEIGHTS AND MEASURES

There is a veritable maze of jargon around marijuana measurements: it can be sold by weight or by the price of the bag, and you've really got to learn the lingo if you want to get the amount you had in mind—and not pay too much for it.

If you're buying your marijuana by weight, you'll usually be buying by ounce—except when you're buying by the metric gram. Standard measurements are, from smallest to largest: a gram to a half-eighth, or sixteenth (⅟₁₆ oz or 1.75g)—the smallest amounts of weed you can buy, and enough for a few mild joints or one fat blunt—an eighth (⅛ oz or 3.5g), a quarter or "quad" (¼ oz or 7g), a half (½ oz or 14g), and an ounce (just over 28g) otherwise known as an "O" or a "zip". At the upper levels, you could by a pound of weed, which is 16 oz (448 g), or a "key" or kilo—and I want to be invited to that party!

To make matters more confusing, you can also buy by the price of a bag. A dime bag costs $10 and should buy you about half a gram; double that, or a "dub" is $20. If you're getting less than a gram for $20 you're probably being ripped off. Never buy three dubs because you can get an eight for a "50 piece"—a.k.a. $50. A quarter (1/4 oz) should set you back roughly $100 and a lid is roughly worth $200, and is often the largest amount a dealer will sell at a time. The term describes the earlier practice of estimating the measurement by simply filling up a tobacco tin all the way to the top (or, to the lid). As in "let's go score a lid."

Note that prices will always vary according to your location, dealer, and the quality of the bud, so a dub sack of low-grade "Schwag" might mean you get 2–3 grams, whereas some hi-grade green may only be one gram.

HEROES OF HEMP: CYPRESS HILL

EVERYONE KNOWS RAPPERS love a nice toke, but the members of Cypress Hill took their love of green to new highs. With classic songs like *Hits from the Bong*, *Insane in the Brain*, *I Wanna Get High*, *K.U.S.H.*, *Ganja Bus*, *Stoned is the Way of the Walk*, *Dr. Greenthumb*, and cover versions of *I Love You Mary Jane* and *Legalise It* all dedicated to their favorite herb, there's no doubting where the West Coast rappers stand on the marijuana debate.

The Latino rock hip-hoppers—currently consisting of DJ Mugs, B Real, Sen Dog, and Eric Bobo—became the officially recognized spokesmen for the National Organization to Reform Marijuana Laws (NORML) back in 1991. They even set up their own successful pro-cannabis Smokeout Music Festival in San Bernardino, California in 1998, which is meant to cater specifically to medical marijuana patients.

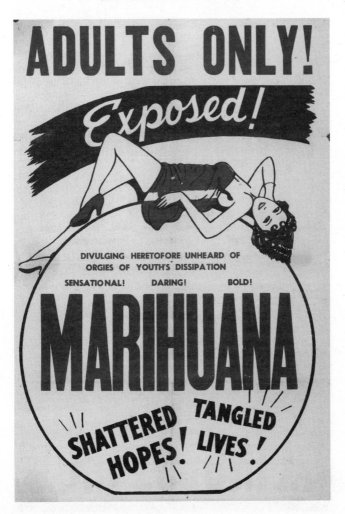

> "When I was in England, I experimented with marijuana a time or two, and I didn't like it and didn't inhale and never tried it again."
> BILL CLINTON, *Former US President (b. 1946)*

GUERRILLA GARDENING

A FRAID OF GROWING GRASS in the garage and getting grabbed by the cops? A safer alternative is guerrilla gardening! Marijuana is a strong, hardy plant that grows practically everywhere—it's not called "weed" for nothing! This makes it ideal for planting in those out-of-the-way hidden places that no one ever goes to, like deep woods or uncultivated fields in the middle of nowhere. The advantage of this is that no one can connect you with the crop unless you're caught harvesting it. The disadvantage is that any stoner can come along and steal it, or worse, the cops could confiscate it. This happened on August 24, 2013, when British police discovered 90 plants growing in the heart of the Norfolk Broads' 116-square mile National Park. However, as PC Paul Bassham pointed out, "In June last year 60 plants were found growing in an area off the River Bure close to Ranworth Broad." Once grass starts to self-seed, it's very hard to get rid of!

Some cheeky guerrilla gardeners have even gone so far as to sow the seeds of dissent in public flower beds outside police stations. If you're going to protest, say it with flowers!

"But let me get to the point, let's roll another joint."
TOM PETTY, *Musician (1950–2017)*

——— WEEDTUBERS: THE STONED STARS ———
OF THE INTERNET

YOUTUBE IS ONE OF THOSE THINGS that feel like they were made for stoners. What did we do before YouTube provided us with stupid videos on tap? Probably went outside and threw rocks at things, or something. One of the great things YouTube has given us is virtual stoner buddies: a whole crop of "WeedTubers" recording themselves getting high, just for our education and entertainment—so you'll never need to smoke alone again! Here are some of our favorite channels:

1. **TokinGLX:** Paul Tokin is a legendary WeedTuber. He's been blazing online since 2006 and is pretty much the classic stoner. He seems like such a nice guy, you know you're in for a chilled one when you're smoking with him. Great if you like nature.

2. **Strain Hunters:** If you like your hits feature-length and kinda epic, follow the crew from Amsterdam's premier coffee shop Green House Seeds as they travel the world on a mission of discovery and education.

3. **Cannabis Longly:** Sometimes we all need to laugh at ourselves, and Cannabis Longly nails some of the commonest problems for stoners – from whether you can resist sparking for 30 minutes until your friend arrives; to the harsh reality of the wake 'n' bake.

5. **SilencedHippie:** Representing a new generation of stoners, Sasha (AKA SilencedHippie) is great company with her chilled vibe and personal touch.

6. **RuffHouse Studios:** A little less blazed and a little more informative than your average WeedTube channel, RuffHouse Studios is a hub for cannabis culture with a huge catalogue of how-to videos to educate you on everything from growing marijuana to the best way of eating it.

7. **CustomGrow420:** Doing it for the love, Joel Hradecky is one glutton for punishment with videos like "1 GRAM DAB CHALLENGE (WARNING DRIPPAGE)" where the suffering is SO REAL. But usually he seems like such a happy guy, and he's one of the most popular WeedTubers out there.

8. **Kimmy Tan:** Kimmy Tan makes smoking weed look super glamorous, but aside from some miraculous makeup skills that keeps her eyeliner looking perfect during "I TRIED TO SMOKE LIKE SNOOP DOGG FOR A DAY"—her most popular video to date—her channel is also full of helpful smoking tips.

— HASH —

THE DARK BLOCKS of what is known as hash originated in India and the Arab world as early as The Bronze Age (think 3000–1000 BCE) and were used as a medicine, either eaten or smoked in a pipe. The name derives from the Arabic for grass (hashish) and is also known as Charas in the Sub-continent. Today hash often goes by the name of its origin and color, such as Lebanese Red, Afghani Black, or Moroccan Brown. The different colors depend on the types of farming, manufacture, and ways of storing it. Hash slowly loses its THC content over time, as it oxidizes, so the fresher the better!

—— MEDICAL MARIJUANA, BIG PHARMA, ——
& THE ENDOCANNABINOID SYSTEM

A S WE SAW EARLIER, CANNABIS has been known for its medical efficacy for thousands of years, but it wasn't until the early '90s that the endocannabinoid system (ECS) was discovered and researchers began to understand why cannabis is so good at treating such a wide variety of illnesses. The main role of the ECS seems to be homeostasis of the body, and so it has receptors all over the body, embedded in different systems, including the immune and the nervous systems. When cannabinoids bind to receptors it's like a switch being flicked to activate a different function, appropriate to the site they're found.

THC, probably the best-known cannabinoid and the one responsible for marijuana's psychoactive effects, for example, has been shown to work with the gastrointestinal system to increase appetite and reduce nausea, a significant benefit to AIDS and cancer patients. Cannabinoids like THC and CBD are also known to be effective at relieving pain, reducing inflammation, suppressing tremors and muscle spasms, inhibiting cancer growth, improving mood and calming anxiety, promoting neurogenesis, and many other therapeutic effects that reduce suffering and help treat problems.

With so many benefits discovered in the relatively short time since marijuana research began to be taken seriously, it's unsurprising that the big pharmaceutical companies are now extracting THC-derivatives and putting it into pills. In 2005 GW Pharmaceuticals brought out a cannabinoid mouth spray called Sativex that relieves pain and spasticity in MS patients. Yet while no one has fatally overdosed from smoking grass, one FDA-approved THC-laden pill, Marinol, has been linked to nasty side effects, including several deaths. Mark Kleiman, director of the Drug Policy Analysis Program at UCLA's School of Public Affairs said, "It [Marinol] wasn't any fun and made the user feel bad, so it could be approved without any fear that it would penetrate the recreational market, and then used as a club with which to beat back the advocates on the whole cannabis as a medicine."

> "Penalties against possession of a drug should not be more
> damaging to an individual than the use of the drug itself…
> Nowhere is this more clear than in the laws against possession
> of marijuana in private for personal use."
>
> JIMMY CARTER, *Former US President (b. 1924)*

"[Marijuana] is not a drug. It's a leaf."
ARNOLD SCHWARZENEGGER, *Actor and Politician (b. 1947)*

MIDNIGHT EXPRESS

ON OCTOBER 7, 1970 an American student, Billy Hayes, was caught trying to smuggle four pounds (2kg) of hashish out of Turkey and was sentenced to four years in prison. His sentence was extended to a life sentence, and then subsequently reduced to 25 years. He eventually escaped İmralı Prison on October 2, 1975 in a rowboat and managed to get over the border to Greece. He recounted his harrowing incarceration in the book, *Midnight Express*, which was turned into a 1978 award-winning film, written by Oliver Stone and directed by Alan Parker. In the film, Hayes discusses his arrest with a shadowy American representative known as "Tex":

Billy Hayes: I didn't have heroin. It was just a little hashish.
Tex: That doesn't matter. A drug's a drug.
Billy Hayes: It was only two kilos.
Tex: It doesn't matter if it was two kilos or 200 kilos. The Turks love catching foreigners. They want to show the rest of the world that they're fighting the drug trade.

The film was criticized for being overly sensational, brutal, and for unfairly portraying Turkey in a particularly bad light. Hayes felt bad about this and eventually returned to the country in 2007—speaking at a conference held by the Turkish National Police—and apologized to the Turkish people.

ACRONYM: THC

Tetrahydrocannabinol is the holy grail of cannabis growing. While there are well over 60 cannabinoids naturally occurring in marijuana, each having a different effect on the human brain, THC is one of the most psychoactive, and is the one that gives stoners that buzz they're all looking for. The highest concentrations of THC are found on the trichome tips of the plant—the sticky resin that is formed. First discovered in 1964, THC causes relaxation, altered vision, hearing, and smell, and increases appetite (AKA "munchies"). But too much *may* induce paranoia and mental problems in developing brains. Interestingly, another cannabinoid, CBD, counteracts many of these problems and so it appears that weed is self-regulating. Oh and it apparently makes male mice sterile, so lay off, Mickey!

ALICE B. TOKLAS

HISTORY'S BEST-KNOWN CANNABIS COOK, Alice B. Toklas, was Gertrude Stein's lover, confidante, and chef. She wrote her 1954 literary memoir, *The Alice B. Toklas Cookbook*, mixing memories with recipes, the most famous being "Haschich Fudge," a blend of fruit, nuts, spices, and cannabis. Technically, this was the North African stoner snack, mahjoun, rather than the hash brownies that she would become linked to. Ironically, Toklas didn't actually come up with the recipe herself, but was given it by her friend Brion Gysin who'd picked it up while in Morocco with William S. Burroughs. Its inclusion in the book was allegedly accidental and a joke, but it caused a sensation. In the book Toklas describes it as "the food of paradise" and hints at where one might score some weed, but like any sensible sinsemilla chef, warns that two pieces are enough to induce hysterical fits of laughter and wild floods of thoughts on "many simultaneous planes." Her infamy was sealed with the title of the 1968 Peter Sellers' film, *I Love You Alice B. Toklas*, which used hash brownies as a major plot device.

WILL WEED
SAVE THE WORLD?

ASIDE FROM BEING A MIND-EXPANDING DRUG that makes music sound better and food more delicious—oh and the many proven medical benefits—cannabis is truly a miracle herb. The Founding Fathers knew this and were strong advocates of cannabis as a crop, long before demonization banished hemp for our fields. These days, more and more people are coming round to its benefits. Here are some of the top reasons why:

- IT CAN FEED THE WORLD. The clue is in the name: weed is a rugged plant that can grow in conditions other crops can't. It has great nutritional content and can be cultivated where food sources are scarce.
- IT MAKES A GREAT BUILDING MATERIAL. "Hempcrete" is a mixture of hemp and lime. It naturally insulates, and it's been claimed the lime in the blended mixture actually grows harder over time, so walls strengthen with age rather than weakening.
- IT CAN REPLACE DESTRUCTIVE MATERIALS. Before cannabis was outlawed, hemp was used in a huge variety of materials, like paper and clothing, that were subsequently replaced by synthetics and other crops. These days, researchers say it could be a biodegradable alternative to oil-based plastics, and a powerful biofuel too.
- IT'S EASIER ON THE LAND. Because cannabis is so tough, it requires far fewer pesticides and herbicides than comparable crops like cotton and wheat, and produces a much higher yield per hectare. Being so nutrient-rich, it can actually improve soil quality.

At the moment, almost all of our hemp is imported from China. Growing it in the U.S. would reduce the cost of importing it—both in terms of money and our carbon footprint.

So should the fields of America be turning green? We think so.

"Dope will get you through times of no money better than money will get you through times of no dope."
GILBERT SHELTON *Freewheelin' Franklin in*
The Fabulous Furry Freak Brothers *(1972)*

——— ETYMOLOGY: TOKE (VERB) ———

Inhaling a small amount marijuana cigarette or pipe smoke. US slang (circa 1952), possibly derived from the Spanish word, *tocar*, meaning "touch, tap, hit" or "get a shave or part."

——————— HEMP FOR VICTORY ———————

THIS US PUBLIC INFORMATION FILM was made in 1942 at a time when resources were low due to the Second World War. It actively encouraged farmers to grow industrial hemp as a means of producing rope, paper, and canvas. After the war the film was forgotten about (or suppressed, if you're a conspiracy fan) until 1989, when activists Jack Herer, Maria Farrow, and Carl Packard finally managed to uncover a recording of it on some old VHS tapes and donated them to the Library of Congress. This wasn't the first time US farmers were encouraged to grow hemp (400,000lbs of seeds were distributed). The first president of the USA, George Washington, grew it and famously wrote, "Make the most you can of the Indian Hemp seed and sow it everywhere." *Popular Mechanics* ran an article in February, 1938 entitled, *New Billion Dollar Crop*, stating, "…The connection of hemp as a crop and marijuana seems to be exaggerated. The drug is usually produced from wild hemp or locoweed, which can be found on vacant lots and along railroad tracks in every state. If federal regulations can be drawn to protect the public without preventing the legitimate culture of hemp, this vast new crop can add immeasurably to American agriculture and industry." Obviously, they couldn't. *Hemp for Victory* was eventually adapted into a 1993 underground comic by Art Penn.

Chronique

Plate 28   *Preparing Hemp II*

Vol. I, Oeconomie rustique, Culture et Travail du Chanvre, Pl. II.

——SUBURBAN SINSEMILLA PRODUCTION——

IN THE UNITED KINGDOM, where cannabis is still illegal, it's estimated that 50% of all cannabis grown in the country is home grown in "factories" or "farms." These are often in unassuming suburban houses that have had six months' rent paid in cash in advance. On moving day, all the furnishings are typically stripped out and vast hydroponic weed beds are installed. The amount of strong lighting and irrigation required for indoor growth generates huge and noticeable levels of thermal radiation (heat), which gives them away to police using thermal-imaging cameras. Another clue that's a red flag is an excessive electricity bill, which can be well over £400 ($490) per month. Many growers bypass this by tapping directly into the electricity supply, with the added danger of house fires. In 2006, in London alone, 50 farms were discovered after catching fire.

Unfortunately, many of these farms are run by criminal gangs that use illegal immigrant child labor to manage their farms. So make sure your supply is ethically sourced! Gangs often grow a single crop for three months and then move to another property, keeping one step ahead of the narcs and leaving the landlords with a devastated property. As one home grower, "Jimmy," explained to the BBC in 2008, "It's a big shame that the organized gangs are taking over. They don't believe in cannabis—to them it's just a way to make money."

Despite all these risks, it's still cheaper and safer for wholesale growers to produce the home-grown stuff than smuggle cannabis into the country from abroad.

IDEAL WEED ON TV

SMOKIN' AND TOKIN' POPS UP all the time in TV shows, from *Shameless* to *Mad Men*, but there have been two outstanding series that have focused exclusively on dope dealers, both of which ran for almost the same length of time. In *Weeds* (2005–2012), Nancy Botwin (played by Mary-Louise Parker) is a widowed Californian suburban housewife who turns to dealing grass to cope financially after her husband's sudden death leaves her family on the brink of bankruptcy. The show follows Nancy's journey from setting up a dealership, finding a client base, and eventually moving on to grow her own supply, and creating her own strain of weed called MILF (slang abbreviation for Mom I'd Like to F**k)! Despite the potentially controversial subject matter, the show was a critical and commercial success, winning a Golden Globe and two Emmys.

In the UK, Graham Duff's darkly surreal sitcom, *Ideal* (get it?) starred Johnny Vegas as Moz, an agoraphobic weed merchant, and focused on the bizarre clients that popped by his Salford flat to score a lid. Running from 2005 until 2011, the storylines featured everything from necrophilia and deadly hit men to killer triads and a character with a mouse mask superglued to his face, known only as "Cartoon Head." Duff explained, "Moz isn't a big player in the world of drugs—far from it. Despite his profession, he actually has principles and won't deal in anything other than cannabis…As a hash dealer, Moz only sees snatches of people's lives—the bits they choose to parade in front of him—but he doesn't see the truth of these people." Duff continued, "The drugs are just a dramatic device. *Ideal* isn't about drugs, it's about the people who have this one thing in common and how their lives interact due to their shared need." Indeed, Moz sees himself as "providing a crucial service to the community." Throughout series five and six Moz gives up dealing, but he eventually returns to selling grass by the final series.

Both TV shows hit a particular zeitgeist, and while both were very dark comedy/dramas, each had a particular idiosyncratic feel relevant to their settings.

CHARAS: A JOINT OPERATION

THIS 2004 BOLLYWOOD ACTION FLICK had British Asian, Dev Anand (Jimmy Shergill) teaming up with an undercover Indian cop (Uday Chopra) to bust marijuana and opium drug barons in the infamous growing valleys of the Ladakh region of India. The convoluted plot twists and turns as Dev searches for his missing botanist pal, Sam, and it is a pretty good film if you can get over the obligatory song and dance numbers.

ETYMOLOGY: BLUNT (NOUN)

This is street slang for "marijuana and tobacco cigar," which started being used in the US around 1993, but is thought to have originated as early as the eighties among Jamaicans in New York City. The term is based on the Phillies Blunt brand cigars, which produce a sweeter smoke. The leaf wrapper of a Phillies Blunt is strong enough to hold together through the process of making a blunt, which involves cutting open and removing the cigar's interior and filling it with weed. However, these days it's much simpler to buy cognac- and honey-dipped tobacco leaves, ready for rolling a nice fat blunt. Can also be used as an adjective—"I got blunted" as in stoned or wasted.

"They've outlawed the number one vegetable on the planet."
TIMOTHY LEARY, *Psychologist and Writer (1920-1996)*

HANDY HEMP

POSSIBLY THE MOST VERSATILE PLANT crop on the planet, hemp has over 50,000 different uses. In the 1800s, and earlier, hemp was one of the most prolific crops used in the industrial manufacture of rope and ships' canvas sails and was a common livestock feed. Even vintage Levi's jeans were made with 40 percent hemp fiber. These days industrial hemp is grown on over 600,000 acres around the world—from Germany and Romania to China—and is used to make beer, flour, cooking oil, and numerous non-intoxicating foods. It makes excellent clothing, soaps, shampoos, sunblock, skateboards, housing materials, and paper products. It has even been extruded into a biodegradable plastic to make bags and CD cases. The Hemp Industries Association (HIA) was established in 1992 to promote and campaign for the fair and equal treatment of hemp in commercial use in North America.

"The mo' dedicated the mo' medicated."
SNOOP DOGG, *Musician (b. 1971)*

──── HEROES OF HEMP: JOE ROGAN ────

JOE ROGAN IS ONE OF THOSE annoying people who can do pretty much anything. He's an actor, a martial artist, a comedian, a writer, a producer, a television host, and a sports commentator. Suffice it to say, this guy gets around. But what we're most concerned with here are his activities as a marijuana user and legalization activist.

This Tae Kwon Do champion and Jiu-Jitsu black belt has been a very vocal champion of the positive effects and benefits of smoking weed for years, both from medical and spiritual standpoints. Though he didn't start properly smoking until he was around thirty (he started late because he bought into the hype that it's a gateway drug and will make you stupid like so many of us), he mostly views marijuana as a spiritual aid, something to clear his head, increase focus and concentration, and help him get in touch with himself. He's also stated that he's found success using it as a workout tool, which, considering how much of a pain fitness can be, is no surprise.

But Rogan does more than just smoke weed, he also evangelizes it. He starred in the 2007 documentary, *The Union: The Business Behind Getting High*, about marijuana prohibition, which likens the war on drugs in this instance to alcohol prohibition in the 1920s, complete with attendant rises in organized crime and lengthy sentences for simple personal possession. Rogan also presented the History Channel documentary *Marijuana: A Chronic History* and has appeared on Marijuana Marketing TV on YouTube. Rogan will often take weed's detractors head on in an erudite debate, blinding them with science and anecdotes of his own personal (positive) experiences with the drug—one of his finest moments was verbally bitch-slapping Dr. Drew for spreading the ridiculous notion that marijuana is addictive and a gateway drug to bath salts (?!). For his tireless advocacy on behalf of our herbal friend, and his ability to talk twice as fast as a normal human, Joe Rogan takes a trophy.

> "Our federal government prohibited this organic plant based on lies, continues to classify it among the most dangerous drugs to validate billions in funding pointless agendas, and denies its medical value, causing countless lives to suffer needlessly. How can anyone not care?"
>
> ROB VAN DAM, *American Pro Wrestler (active 1990–Present)*

CANNABUTTER

THERE'S MORE TO COOKING with weed than just chucking a bunch of leaves and buds into a pot and stirring. If you really want to get that buzz you've got to release the active ingredient, Tetrahydrocannabinol (THC), from the plant. Because THC isn't water soluble, you need to break it down in fats or oil and the best way to do this is to make cannabutter or ghee. Here's how to make the former:

1 You'll need 1–2lbs (0.5–1kg) of butter and 2–3oz (55–85g) of finely ground/powdered marijuana tops or buds. This should make more than enough for several recipes.

2 Melt the butter on a low heat and then add the grass. Simmer slowly until the butter turns a greenish color. Be careful not to burn the butter as that will ruin the flavor and destroy the THC. "Slow and low" is best.

3 Next, strain the butter through a very fine sieve or muslin and set the leafy material aside.

4 If you really want to up the potency of the butter you can repeat steps 1–3 with a bunch of fresh marijuana, but go easy, cannabis in cooking takes twice as long as a joint to cause a high, but it is twice as strong! So always err on the side of caution.

5 When the cannabutter has cooled you can refrigerate or freeze and use as needed. It's a good idea to pour a little water over the top, which seals it for freshness.

6 The leftover leafy material can be simmered in hot milk and sweetened with honey to make a delicious dope drink. Just remember to take it easy!

—————————— HERB VS. "HERB" ——————————

THE RELATIONSHIP BETWEEN marijuana and dried oregano is as long as it is contentious. There are many documented (and tragic) cases of unscrupulous dealers selling innocuous old oregano to newbies in the guise of weed. What's more, there's also no shortage of anecdotes of those same amateurs later smoking their top-quality oregano and either pretending or believing they're toking the real reefer (belief is a powerful thing). The confusion is understandable to a point; while the two dried plants share the same dirty green hue and do look similar from a distance (dealers will often wrap the fake weed up well in semi-transparent plastic), the real divider is the smell. If your herb smells like it belongs in an Italian restaurant, don't try to smoke it. If it has a top-note of skunk (the animal—hence the variety name), you're probably in possession of the real thing. It's perfectly acceptable to take a whiff of the product before making a purchase, and at the end of the day, practice makes perfect.

(On a related note, tomato plants are sometimes mistaken for pot plants, so be sure to keep interfering neighbors away from your legal vegetable garden.)

> "The only effect that I ever noticed from smoking marijuana was a sort of mild sedative, a release of tension when I was overworking."
>
> ROBERT MITCHUM, *Actor (1917–1997)*

——— TOP 15 DOPEST HIP-HOP TUNES ———

These rappers are all about the chronic:

1 *High All Time* BY 50 CENT (*Get Rich or Die Tryin'*, 2003)

2 *Get High Tonight* BY BUSTA RHYMES (*When Disaster Strikes*, 1997)

3 *Pack The Pipe* BY THE PHARCYDE (*Bizarre Ride II the Pharcyde*, 1992)

4 *Indo Smoke* BY MISTER GRIMM (*Poetic Justice Soundtrack*, 1983)

5 *Tical* BY METHOD MAN (*Tical*, 1994)

6 *How High* BY REDMAN AND METHOD MAN (*The Blackout*, 1999)

7 *I Can't Wake Up* BY KRS-ONE (*Return of the Boom Bap*, 1993)

8 *How to Roll a Blunt* BY REDMAN (*Whut? Thee Album*, 1992)

9 *Doobie Ashtray* BY DEVIN THE DUDE (*Just Tryin' ta Live*, 2002)

10 *Weed Song* BY BONE THUGS-N-HARMONY (*BTNHresurrection*, 2000)

11 *I Wanna Get High* BY CYPRESS HILL (*Black Sunday*, 1993)

12 *Cheeba Cheeba* BY TONE LOC (*Loc-ed After Dark*, 1989)

13 *Smoke Some Weed* BY ICE CUBE (*Laugh Now, Cry Later*, 2006)

14 *Down 2 tha Last Roach* BY EAZY-E (*It's On (Dr. Dre) 187um Killa*, 1993)

15 *The Roach* BY DR. DRE (*The Chronic*, 1992)

A MOMENT OF SILENCE
FOR THE LESS FORTUNATE

ONE COULD BE FORGIVEN FOR ASSUMING this book has come down on the pro-marijuana side of the great pot debate, mostly because it has. We've discussed the medicinal value of pot, both scientifically proved and anecdotally suggested; the value of hemp to industry and environment; reasons for its prohibition; reasons for and against medical and general legalization; how to roll a joint; recipes; and basically just how fun the stuff is…for most people. But weed has a little-discussed dark side that even its most determined advocates cannot deny.

Cannabis is a drug, but first and foremost, it's a plant. More specifically, it's a flowering herb. Despite marijuana's medical benefits, between ten and 30 percent of the world's population may be excluded from using this wondrous drug because of a single side effect: allergies. That's right: standard, run-of-the-mill, summer-is-hell-kill-me-now-oh-god pollen and plant allergies.

While marijuana allergies haven't been investigated in depth, some people have reported skin rashes, hives, rhinitis, flu-like symptoms, and breathing problems after indulging. This is hardly surprising given the plant connection and experts believe that marijuana allergies might be more common than previously assumed. In 2011, Dr. Gordon Sussman, acting division director of clinical allergy and immunology at the University of Toronto, conducted a study of 17 patients who complained of allergic reactions following cannabis use and all 17 tested positive for sensitivity following skin-prick tests. One patient experienced anaphylactic shock from drinking marijuana tea. The causes and mechanics of the allergies aren't well known and probably won't be any time soon; it's difficult to conduct proper studies on illegal drugs, even in clinical and academic environments, and marijuana allergies are most likely drastically under reported because patients are (understandably) reluctant to confess illegal drug use to their doctors.

Do not condemn these unfortunate individuals, fair reader; do not laugh or jeer at this profound disability. Instead, treat them as they deserve to be treated—with pity. They deserve our sympathy and compassion.

HIP-HOP HEMPSTERS

THIS CATEGORY OF SMOKER is densely populated. Not only is marijuana use and reference rife in hip-hop culture, it's at the level of being almost a badge of honor. These are some of our favorite musical icons who also happen to be massive stoners.

1 Method Man and Redman
Rap's finest comedy duo has what could accurately be called prolific smoking habits and they aren't afraid to tweet the visual evidence. Their music, both as solo artists and a team, is filled with references to their favorite pastime— witness *How High*, *A Special Joint*, and *Dis Iz 4 All My Smokers* among many, many others—and they even starred in their own ill-reviewed but cult favorite stoner film *How High* (2001). We want them to be our best friends.

2 Cypress Hill
With titles like *I Love You Mary Jane*, *Roll It Up*, *Light It Up*, *Smoke It Up*, and *K.U.S.H.*, most Cypress Hill tracks read like love letters to weed, and their songs regularly appear on lists of the best songs to get high by. Their rep is further fueled by the fact that they have an uncanny ability to sound like smoking feels.

3 Snoop Dogg
Snoop Dogg is the incarnate existence of herbal celebration. He smokes it, he loves it, he lives it. The music connections are obvious, but he often shows up as the pimping and/or pot-loving minor character when needed in movies and TV shows. We even liked his horror anthology movie *Hood of Horror* (2002) just because he was in it, even though it really wasn't very good and isn't the kind of thing you want to watch while smoking.

4 Curren$y
Smoking weed isn't just something this New Orleans native does; it's an integral part of his whole public (and we're betting private) identity. All of the references in his music are there, but he's also an outspoken smoker outside of his lyrics. He's also been known to give advice to fellow enthusiasts; according to Curren$y, blunts are expensive and bad for you, so stick to papers.

5 Wiz Khalifa
This man isn't just a weed smoker, he's a *connoisseur*. This man has his own strain of marijuana, Khalifa Kush, which was cultivated for him according to his taste and personal high preferences. But don't go looking for it at your medical dispensary or (legal) recreational shop just yet—it's still too rare for general consumption.

—— POTUMENTARIES ——

Amidst the many silly-ass fiction movies that revolve around smoking-related high jinx and the anti-marijuana propaganda films masquerading as nonfiction, there are some pretty informative films on the market for anyone looking for less negative and/or more scientific views of the herb. Here are five documentaries we recommend for education rather than entertainment (some of which are available in their entirety on YouTube):

1 In Pot We Trust (2007) This pro-pot film takes a look at legalization in the US and features arguments from both sides of the aisle. Through interviews with academics, politicians, and political lobbyists, the police, DEA officials, and medical marijuana users (including those specifically supplied by the federal government—that's right: *federal*, not state), *In Pot We Trust* intersperses personal stories of those who've been helped by marijuana for medical use. If you're already pro-legalization for medical use, it'll be preaching to the converted, but those on the fence or in the anti camp may have their eyes opened a little to pot's benefits for those who suffer.

2 The Union: The Business Behind Getting High (2007) Featuring the well known Hero of Hemp, Joe Rogen, *The Union* is staunchly and unabashedly pro-legalization and it makes an excellent case. Through a brief history lesson, comparisons to alcohol prohibition, and expert and enthusiast interviews, the film attempts to prove that the war on drugs began as a war on marijuana in the 1970s, intended to stamp out political unrest, specifically Vietnam War protests. The resultant anti-drug machine has become such big business with so many tentacles that it's in the government's (and many private sectors') best interest to keep marijuana illegal. It's a fairly depressing outlook on the legalization of weed in the US, but an essential educational tool.

3 Grass: The History of Marijuana (1999) Narrated by noted pothead Woody Harrelson, *Grass* chronicles the troubled history of marijuana in the USA, starting with its link to Mexican laborers and progressing through to Anslinger's involvement and decades of government anti-drug propaganda. The film is more colorful and lighthearted than the other docs on this list, but its message is still clear: The US government's marijuana policy is misguided and harmful to the American public.

4 Super High Me (2007) Comedian and pothead Doug Benson takes the Morgan Spurlock challenge, but with marijuana: he spends 30 days not smoking at all, followed by 30 days of smoking all day, every day. Benson takes physical and mental tests both while smoking and sober, for comparison, and the results are surprising, if not groundbreaking. Benson's story is peppered with the processes and plights of medical dispensaries in California, and includes an interview with Hero of Hemp Marc Emery.

5 Marijuana Inc.: Inside America's Pot Industry (2009) Produced by CNBC, this doc investigates the pot industry in northern California, from legal growing to smuggling, and its effects on the local culture and economy. It's remarkably evenhanded for having been produced by one of the major US news networks, but highlights the difficulty and consequences of growing in a legal state where federal laws still outlaw cultivation and consumption.

—————— THE BIG APPLE BONG ——————

EARLY IN 2014, New York State governor Andrew Cuomo announced he would allow limited use of marijuana for medical reasons (marijuana had previously been illegal for all uses). On the one hand, we wonder what took so long for such a purportedly liberal state that includes New York City, that bastion of excess and hedonism, among its constituents to get on the weed bandwagon. On the other hand, Cuomo has historically opposed medical marijuana, New York State still has the death penalty, and NYC has proved enough of a nanny city to ban e-cigarettes in public and require all chain restaurants to post calorie counts (because otherwise we'd think McDonald's is serving up the elixir of life blended into a McFlurry).

But don't go planning your move to the Big Apple yet—medical marijuana in New York will be tightly controlled and restricted for use only in a handful of hospitals and by the seriously ill, so insomnia and occasional tension headaches won't get you a weed card like those California hippies. But don't despair: in a larger sense, New York is now the twenty-first state in the US to legalize medical marijuana, which is just another step toward universal acceptance.

> "Look, when I was a kid, I inhaled. Frequently. That was the point."
> BARACK OBAMA, *US President (b. 1961)*

POT PENS

CANNABIS VAPORIZERS HAVE BEEN on the market for ages, but they've always been relatively expensive and unwieldy. Classic, cone-shaped vaporizers can run to hundreds of dollars, but many smokers prefer them as they provide a healthier alternative to lighting the weed on fire and dragging the particulates into their lungs. Used with either buds or oil, vaporizers give a stronger high with less damage to both the source material and the smoker. But they've never been a particularly portable alternative to smoking, and this is where e-cigarettes have come in to lend a bit of technological innovation to their less-legal brother.

Like traditional cigarettes, e-cigarettes were designed to be carried around and puffed at will, aping the "oh my god I need something to do with my hands and what about my oral fixation" habit of the daily smoker (one of the many reasons that patches, inhalers, and cold-turkey quitting fail so often—they don't satisfy the *act* of smoking, just the nicotine addiction). So lo and behold the e-cigarette was born and it's amazing. The device, in its most basic sense, works by heating up a mixture of liquid nicotine and a carrier agent (often propylene glycol) to create a vapor that can be inhaled. It wasn't long before some intrepid young potheads noticed that the e-cigarette device could be applied to "smoking"—properly termed vaping—hash oil as well. The original technology needed to be modified as you can't just pour some oil into a standard e-cigarette and achieve the desired results—although there are hacks available—but there are now pens on the market that look and act very much like e-cigarettes and can be used with oils, waxes, and dry herb. Of course, this stealth ability just may be their undoing, as twitchy lawmakers are starting to realize that, in public, it's hard to tell the difference between someone legally vaping nicotine and illegally vaping cannabis. Only time will tell whether this new technology will be "regulated" into oblivion by the THINK OF THE CHILDREN! brigade, so there may be only a limited time in which to buy devices to vape the reefer. Go forth and conquer.

HEROES OF HEMP: MARC EMERY

POPULARLY KNOWN AS "The Prince of Pot," Marc Emery has shown his activist chops in a variety of ways, from leading a legalization-platform political party to supplying paraphernalia and seeds to the people. This guy has done just about everything he can in the name of weed.

Originally from London, Ontario in Canada, Emery demonstrated an entrepreneurial spirit early on by forming mail-order businesses before he even went through puberty. If that doesn't make you feel inadequate enough, he bought and ran a bookshop while he was still a teenager, and then started to participate seriously in local politics in his early twenties. He clearly had a problem with government censorship and "nanny state" intervention, as he would sell banned albums and literature (including *High Times* magazine) specifically to contravene Canadian law.

After moving to Vancouver in the mid-nineties, Emery opened a head shop, which was a bit of a problem as it was illegal to sell drug paraphernalia and literature in Canada at the time. At this point, he'd more than proved his willingness to break laws he didn't agree with, which makes him sound like a bit of a jerk, but his end game was nobler than it seemed. Emery soon sponsored a case against Canada's laws prohibiting the sale of paraphernalia and literature, and he succeeded in overturning the prohibition. A year later Emery started a marijuana mag of his own: *Cannabis Culture*.

However, Emery's head for business and law-breaking eventually became his downfall. His head shop also sold seeds, and after numerous raids and fines, he switched to mail-order only in the late nineties. As he would ship anywhere in the world, his distribution efforts became an international issue, and in 2005 he was arrested at the request of the US Drug Enforcement Agency for international drug trafficking. Amidst worldwide protests, Emery spent the next five years fighting extradition to the US. He eventually copped a plea and was sentenced to five years in US federal prison.

Marc Emery is one of the most important Heroes of Hemp to emerge out of the past thirty years, because he didn't just use cannabis, talk about how great it is, or make money off it; he also helped bring the legalization issue to worldwide political attention and actually changed the arcane anti-cannabis laws in Canada. Despite raids, fines, arrests, harassment, and ultimately imprisonment, he's remained a staunchly vocal and political supporter of smokers' rights and a hero to decriminalization and legalization movements globally. It's probably a bit of an overstatement to say he's the Gandhi of weed, but Emery has certainly been the change he wished to see in the world.

——————— PAPERS TO READ, NOT ROLL ———————

APPARENTLY POTHEADS LIKE TO READ. A lot. So it's a good thing there are so many sources of information in print and online, giving everything from reviews to advice to techniques and interviews. These are four of the more established magazines available to the discerning weed aficionado today:

1 High Times: No discussion of marijuana-reading material can be considered complete without mentioning *High Times*. First published in 1974, the magazine has become the *Playboy* of pot, complete with a monthly fold-out centerfold (but most people read it for the articles). Willing to change with the times, *High Times* is now available online as well as in print, and in 2010 launched *Medical Marijuana News & Reviews*, a sister publication devoted to medical marijuana activism.

2 Cannabis Culture: Launched in 1995 under the name *Cannabis Canada*, *Cannabis Culture* was founded by Marc Emery, a noted legalization activist, who became the leader of the British Columbia Marijuana Party in 2000. The publication dropped print and became wholly online in 2005, where it provides readers with news and views on the struggle of legalization, as well as growing tips and interviews with cannacelebrities.

3 420 Magazine: This California-based magazine is the largest publication in the US based on the medical marijuana movement and has been preaching to readers since 1993. Its mission is to support the full legalization of cannabis throughout the world, and it does that by educating its readers with facts, news, scientific data, legal information, and an online community forum for like-minded people.

4 Cannabis Now: One of the newer magazines on this list, *Cannabis Now* is devoted almost entirely to the medical marijuana movement. Its prime objective is education, and as such, it's less about celebrity interviews and more dedicated to pieces on responsible consumption; political, economic, and legal news and commentary; and researched-based facts and figures on the drug to combat the hysteria and ignorance that largely prevent legalization.

THE CANNABIS CONSPIRACY

IN THE COMICS WORLD, British artist and writer Bryan Talbot is no joke. He began his career in comics with underground comix in the sixties and progressed to *The Adventures of Luther Arkwright* in the late seventies, the comic series for which he is probably most famous. That was still the beginning of his career, however, and since then he's worked on *Judge Dredd* for 2000 AD, *Sandman* and *Batman* for DC Comics, and *Fables* for Vertigo. His own creations include *Alice in Sunderland*, *Grandville*, *The Tale of One Bad Rat*, and, most relevant to this book, *The Cannabis Conspiracy*.

The Cannabis Conspiracy is only four pages long, but the Eagle and Eisner Award-winning creator packs in quite a bit. Beginning with a short history of marijuana and hemp in America, Talbot posits that the prohibition of cannabis began as a conspiracy orchestrated by William Randolph Hearst, the Dupont family, and Andrew Mellon to ban hemp in favor of their own profitable and patented methods of paper, rope, and cloth manufacture. It all seems a bit hysterical at first—a paranoid fantasy invented by a sixties flower child—but taking a step back, it does make a sick kind of sense. Approaching the marijuana debate from whatever angle you like, it will eventually be distilled down to a matter of money—whether it's the money that flows through the government anti-drug machine, the lack of profit for pharmaceutical companies that have tried and failed for decades to produce an effective synthetic version in light of the fact that plants can't be patented, or the campaign dollars politicians won't receive if they endorse marijuana legalization in their conservative districts. And this doesn't even begin to address the industries that depend on deforestation for their products, and which would probably go out of business if hemp became a legal alternative for creating paper and other saleable fibers.

In light of the current political and financial climate in the US, is it really that farfetched to suggest that cannabis prohibition began as a way for the richest and most powerful men in America to stay rich and powerful? Whether you believe it or not, *The Cannabis Conspiracy* will make you consider that question carefully, and when you're done, you might just need a little weed to lift the depression.

THAT '70S SHOW: MYSTERY SOLVED

REMEMBER THE CIRCLE? Where different combinations of characters would sit around a table and everyone's eyes would be red, they all seemed really chilled out while they chatted, and the air would be suspiciously smoky but you never actually saw what was going on? Turns out they were smoking weed. For real. We're surprised too.

A VAGUE HISTORY OF MEDICAL MARIJUANA

IT SEEMS ODD THAT THE MODERN mainstream public has been so opposed to cannabis for so long, even for medicinal purposes, when the drug has been used as a healing aid by all sections of society, including the most venerated, for the past 5,000 years (that we know of). Let's skip back through history, shall we, and discover what our elders—some may say "betters"—were using this leafy little wonder drug for. You might be surprised how modern their marijuana sensibilities were.

Circa 2700 BC: Chinese Emperor Shen Nung is considered the father of Chinese medicine and is said to have eaten hundreds of herbs to determine whether they had any medicinal properties. Legend has it that he discovered the healing properties of weed and used it to treat pretty much everything, from malaria to diarrhea to (unsurprisingly) vomiting.

2000 to 1400 BC: In India, cannabis was not only used as a spiritual aid, but also as an Ayurvedic remedy to treat insomnia, stress, and indigestion. Later it was purported to be a cure for leprosy.

Circa 1770 BC to 1100 BC: Judging by their medical texts, the Ancient Egyptians loved themselves some herb. They used hemp oil mixed with honey to treat inflammation and pre-menstrual symptoms, as well as crushed up seeds for colorectal issues.

500 BC to first century AD: Medical men of the Greek and Roman persuasion found cannabis quite useful for problems such as earache and nosebleeds, but also used it to (ahem) "dry up the seed" of adolescent boys and warned that excessive use could cause sexual dysfunction.

Fifteenth century: Muslim scholars were faced with a dilemma over marijuana—they recognized its medicinal value, but also its intoxicating qualities, and debated whether it should be treated akin to alcohol, which is expressly forbidden by the Koran. They eventually decided to differentiate between the two uses, allowing medical marijuana, but severely punishing recreational use.

Nineteenth century: Marijuana wasn't widely used in the US and Europe until Irish doctor William O'Shaughnessy conducted his own research into cannabis' medical applications. He used it to treat pain and the often-fatal symptoms of cholera. In 1860, the Ohio State Medical Society held the first American conference on medical marijuana, and found it to be successful in treating gonorrhea and pain, among other afflictions.

Twentieth century: Despite worldwide legality issues, marijuana is strongly indicated in the treatment of chronic pain, side effects from chemotherapy, loss of appetite, and symptoms of AIDS, for example. While not recognized as a cure for any disease, it can greatly increase quality of life in the sick by alleviating symptoms and side effects.

— HEROES OF HEMP: LESTER GRINSPOON —

IF YOU WATCH SOME OF THE POTUMENTARIES listed in this book, you'll recognize Lester Grinspoon. If you're a proponent of medical marijuana, you should know who he is anyway.

Currently an associate professor of psychiatry, emeritus, at Harvard Medical School, Grinspoon saw his friends and contemporaries use marijuana quite a bit during the sixties and, as a doctor, decided to do a little research into this drug he'd heard, and believed, was so harmful. His extensive investigation covered all research available in the Harvard libraries, and he came to believe that marijuana wasn't dangerous at all, despite the hype. At the time he published a book on that lack of danger called *Marihuana Reconsidered* in 1971—which included a pro-pot essay by "Mr. X," also known as Carl Sagan— Grinspoon's teenage son had been suffering the effects of chemotherapy used to treat his leukemia. The worst of it was constant vomiting and lack of appetite. While Grinspoon couldn't endorse his son's use of illegal drugs, his wife procured a little pot for their son to smoke, hoping to alleviate the chemo's side effects. Grinspoon then witnessed first-hand the medical benefits of weed, as his son stopped vomiting and regained his appetite. Though his son didn't make it in the end, Grinspoon believes that the quality of his remaining life was greatly increased by marijuana.

Since then, Grinspoon has wholeheartedly endorsed marijuana's medical applications, prompting scientific studies into its effectiveness as well as personally publishing on its ability to alleviate suffering in those afflicted with numerous diseases. Even though he believes his course of study may have affected the progress of his career, he has remained a vocal and important proponent of the drug, calling for its legalization as a medicine.

> "Marijuana will be legal some day, because the many law students who now smoke pot will someday become Congressmen and legalize it in order to protect themselves."
>
> LENNY BRUCE, *American comedian* (1925–1966)

STONER GAMES

ALTHOUGH BOARD GAMES SEEM to be a thing of the past these days, having been eclipsed by more recent entertainment inventions that beep and blink, and change images every half second, stoners still embrace the cards and dice. Probably because video games move just a bit too fast when you're high. Here are five board and card games that center around bud:

1 Reefer City: Billed as "the game for intelligent heads," Reefer City uses the standard Monopoly format with board, dice, cards, and funny money. The object is to make your way through the city selling weed, hash, and shrooms without getting arrested. It bundles entertainment and useful life skills into one box.

2 Stoner City: Despite the similar title, this one is less imaginative than Reefer City. It's a straight Monopoly rip-off, with the only addition to gameplay being a police car that travels in the opposite direction of the players—when the car and a player land on the same space, the player goes to rehab (Stoner City's highly original version of jail).

3 Stoner Fluxx: Fluxx is almost impossible to play drunk due to the complexity of its rules, so we're not sure how successful it would be to play the stoner version. The rules are basically the same, but with pot-themed cards, you can feel as good about the purchase as the play, because five percent of proceeds go to the Marijuana Policy Project, NORML, and other organizations devoted to legalizing marijuana.

4 The Official Dealer McDope Dealing Game: This game is no longer made, but it was a classic of the 1970s (and you can find it on any auction site or at garage sales). Created by legendary comix artist Dave Sheridan, Dealer McDope involves players buying and selling weed while avoiding prison. The first dealer to reach two million dollars wins. It's a lot to pack in to a board, dice, and a deck of cards.

5 Trafficking: Originally created in the fabulous eighties, Trafficking has its players take on the roles of drug dealers and a Narc. The winner, or "Traffic King," is the first dealer to sell one kilo of marijuana without being arrested by the Narc. Controversial enough to be banned only a few years after it was released, Trafficking is now on the market again and will probably teach you more about business than any Ivy League school.

--- NORML ---

FOUNDED in 1970 by attorney Keith Stroup, the National Organization for the Reform of Marijuana Laws (NORML) is dedicated to the decriminalization of marijuana. It has hundreds of chapters across the United States, as well as partner programs in other countries such as New Zealand, Ireland, and the United Kingdom). The organization also seeks to educate the public on marijuana, contradicting much of the false information disseminated by the government to support the War on Drugs by publishing detailed scholarly work on the subject of marijuana's medicinal use. They maintain an impressive media presence in a variety of venues, from billboards in Times Square, to television commercials, to petitions to the White House. They also use legal tools to keep the pressure on the government—in 1972 NORML sued the Drug Enforcement Administration, arguing for the legalization of medical marijuana. You'll also find their support and grassroots activist groups behind many state's individual decriminalization/legalization legislative pushes. Marijuana has now been decriminalized in some states and legalized in Washington and Colorado, but NORML still has a lot of work to do to achieve its goal of total acceptance. Luckily, it has the help of a star roster of an advisory board, which includes Willie Nelson, Woody Harrelson, Tommy Chong, Bill Maher, Nadine Strossen (president of the ACLU), and, formerly, Robert Altman and Hunter S. Thompson.

—— URUGUAY CROSSES THE FINISH LINE ——

JOSÉ MUJICA, THE PRESIDENT OF URUGUAY, is known to be one of the most liberal politicians on the planet and rivals Pope Francis in the humility and charity departments. He gives about 90 percent of his salary to charity, lives on a farm instead of in the presidential palace, and drives a 25-year-old Volkswagen Beetle. In which case, it really shouldn't have been a surprise when this bleeding-heart hippie legalized marijuana in 2013.

Smoking has been legal in the country for decades, so Uruguay has gone a step further with its new legislation: the state is intent on fully creating, licensing, and regulating a countrywide marijuana industry. Once the law is put into effect, any registered adult will be able to grow weed in their own home, take part in a club to grow as a collective, or buy joints from pharmacies. By bringing control of the drug into state hands, Uruguayan law-makers hope to discourage the illegal drug trade, effectively stripping the cartels of their money and power.

Sounds like a pretty great idea, doesn't it? But the move isn't without its detractors (of course). The United Nations in particular has publicly denounced Uruguay's planned legalization, saying that it could hurt the country's children and contribute to addiction. Apparently the UN hasn't got the memo about cannabis not being a) addictive and b) a gateway drug. But then they probably still use *Reefer Madness* as a documentary/training video.

As much as Uruguay's new law may bode well for legalization, or at least decriminalization, on the international scene in the (distant?) future, and as much as we admire José Mujica's common-sense approach to the War on Drugs despite his personal dislike for recreational chemicals, don't go changing your holiday plans from Amsterdam to Uruguay just yet. The laws are also specifically designed to prevent marijuana tourism, as only registered adults will be able to buy the goods, and only citizens of Uruguay may register. There's no indication whether this will change anytime soon, so for now a weekend getaway to Denver might be in order (out-of-staters can legally buy a quarter of an ounce).

—————— STONER GAMES 2: THE GAMENING ——————

FOR THOSE OF YOU WHO LIKE your gaming action a bit more interactive—more "real," one might say—there are a few video games out there that feature the drug in creative ways. Here are four of the more direct references and one upcoming game that's more of an instructional video:

1 Grand Theft Auto series: Weed has been a minor staple of the *GTA* franchise since the beginning, with many characters indulging in a bit of herb here and there (the main character never smokes himself, but he does deal and run drug missions for others). In *San Andreas*, an entire mission involves burning a weed field for an old hippie voiced by none other than Peter Fonda, which is quite the tribute.

2 Afro Samurai: Originally a manga series that was then adapted to anime, Afro Samurai is, unsurprisingly, a black samurai hell bent on revenge. Although the suspiciously cone-shaped roll-up perpetually hanging out of his mouth isn't explicitly referred to as a joint, have a look and draw your own conclusion. (Bonus evidence: Afro is voiced by Samuel L. Jackson.)

3 Saints Row 1 and 2: *Saints Row* takes the *GTA* casual weed use a bit further by allowing the main character to buy and smoke, but also suffer its effects. While we wouldn't normally equate smoking with suffering, the character control takes a hit from distorted vision and coughing fits.

4 Call of Juarez: The Cartel: Seeing as this is a game based on Mexican drug cartels, it's of no surprise that marijuana should make a prominent showing. The somewhat depressing gameplay involves a shoot out in a marijuana field, and no one gets high. Not much fun, then.

5 GROWsim: At the end of 2013, creator Matt Di Spirito released the Beta version of his indie *GROWsim* "game," which is basically a simulation of how to grow medical marijuana. This doesn't really fit into the entertainment category, but it certainly has educational value, so it may be the most justifiable game on this list to spend money on.

> "Never smoke pot before there's a possibility of talking to a hundred million people."
>
> WHOOPI GOLDBERG, *Actress (b. 1955)*

—— WRITING UNDER THE INFLUENCE ——

A UTHORIAL TYPES HAVE NEVER BEEN strangers to drugs—in fact, they have a bit of a reputation for enjoying the more hedonistic things in life. Some prefer booze, others LSD, but the creators on this list are prime examples of the benefits of writing while baked.

1 Aaron Sorkin
It's not that hard to work out Sorkin's had problems with drugs, as every TV show he writes has at least one recovering-addict-turned-wiseman on the character roster. Autobiographical much? Anyway, his particular cocktail contains, among others, the reefer, which he apparently tokes (or toked) to get his creative juices flowing.

2 Rick Steves
This one's a little unexpected, considering Steves' reputation for being popular with independent travelers of a certain age, but perhaps his soporific demeanor gave us the clue. Steves believes the drug's mind-expanding qualities have made him become a better writer (with more than 20 bestselling guidebooks on the market, he should know). But Steves goes beyond mere use, as he's also a strong advocate of decriminalization, evidenced by his seat on the board of directors of NORML. He also worked on the TV program *Marijuana: It's Time for a Conversation*, which was produced by the ACLU.

3 Stephen King

King is another writer who's had drug problems in the past (let's not be too surprised—writing is a pain in the ass), and much of his work during the eighties doesn't bode well for writers who want to use cocaine as a creative stimulant. Weed, however, is a different story, and King is enough of a fan to advocate legalization.

4 Lee Child

In August 2013, Lee Child, the bestselling author of the Jack Reacher novels, told the *Daily Mail* newspaper that he's "been smoking weed for 44 years, five nights a week." Considering he's on his way to reaching 100 million in book sales, it doesn't seem to have done his writing career any harm and could even be considered an asset.

5 Alexandre Dumas and friends

The author of *The Count of Monte Cristo*, *The Three Musketeers*, and many other stories of romance and adventure liked his hashish and no mistake. Along with Charles Baudelaire, Honoré de Balzac, and Victor Hugo, Dumas was a member of the Club des Hashischins, which was dedicated to exploring mind-altering experiences with drugs like opium and, more often, hashish. While Dumas is perhaps the most populist writer of the group, the one thing all these men have in common is that, more than 100 years after their deaths, they're still widely known and read. Not bad for a bunch of nineteenth-century stoners.

6 Hunter S. Thompson

This entry on the list should be a surprise to exactly nobody, but it has to be said that among all the other drugs Thompson indulged in, marijuana was one of his favorites. He's called it "one of the staples of life," has served on the board of NORML, advocated legalization, and smoked right up to the end of his life because he believed the drug prevented Alzheimer's. And if recent research is anything to go by, he wasn't far off the mark.

7 Carl Sagan

Astrophysicist, author, luminary, pothead. Carl Sagan not only smoked marijuana himself, he advocated its use for its mind-expanding properties, and even contributed an essay to *Marihuana Reconsidered*, published in 1971, using the pseudonym "Mr. X." He wrote that "the illegality of cannabis is outrageous, an impediment to full utilization of a drug which helps produce the serenity and insight, sensitivity and fellowship so desperately needed in this increasingly mad and dangerous world." While his advocacy and use was kept secret until after his death, he still managed to communicate his beliefs on the drug as effectively as those on science.

8 Alan Moore

The author of such groundbreaking comics as *Watchmen*, *V for Vendetta*, *From Hell*, and *Batman: The Killing Joke* is also a massive stoner. In between his duties worshipping Glycon, his snake god, and performing ceremonial magic, Moore smokes what has been termed a "prodigious" amount of weed. According to artist Rick Veitch, "Next time you read one of Alan's extensive interviews in print or online, and are marveling at the fact he is speaking off the cuff like Herman Melville wrote novels on a good day, you can probably be certain the interview was conducted under the influence of enough wacky tobbacky to put Cheech and Chong under the table."

9 William Butler Yeats

Nobel Prize-winning poet Yeats was a keen believer in the occult, going so far as joining the Hermetic Order of the Golden Dawn and the Theosophical Society, both dedicated to mystic ritual and investigation. Of course, mind-expanding activities such as these are often aided by the use of mind-altering drugs, and Yeats began using hashish in pellet form in the 1890s after visiting Paris, that notorious hotbed of cannabactivity. He used the drug to enhance creativity and commune with mystical forces, and considering he won a Nobel, it seems to have worked.

10 Allen Ginsberg

Drugs and the Beat Generation go hand in hand. While Ginsberg and his contemporaries are most known for their use and advocacy of LSD, Ginsberg also supported marijuana legalization. In 1966 he published an essay in *The Atlantic Monthly* called "The Great Marijuana Hoax: First Manifesto to End the Bringdown," which chronicled his own use of the drug while making a case for the absurdity of its illegality. He also mentions that most of the creatives he knows—actors, musicians, writers, artists, poets, and sculptors—have been smoking for decades. Which is pretty much what we've been saying all along.

"Wine makes men happy and sociable; hashish isolates them.
Wine exalts the will; hashish annihilates it."

CHARLES BAUDELAIRE, *Poet (1821–1867)*

—— EAR WAX: IT'LL BLOW YOUR ASS UP ——

EAR WAX is a relative newcomer to the hash scene. Named for its brown, sticky, ear waxy appearance, it's estimated to be anywhere from 50 to 90 percent THC (by contrast, the flower alone is more like five to ten percent). Seems like heaven, one might think, but it's already caused some trouble due to its method of manufacture and its effects.

It's easy to find tutorials on how to make Ear Wax on YouTube, but the most common method seems to be to soak the bud in butane to extract the oil (known as BHO, or butane hash oil), evaporate the butane, and then heat the oil to concentrate it into a thick, golden-brown resin. Seems relatively simple and straightforward, doesn't it? Unfortunately, when cannabis resin production starts to resemble cooking meth, (breaking) bad things are going to happen. So it was with two Brooklyn, New York, teenagers in 2013 who thought it would be a good idea to fill a barrel with butane and then light a cigarette. Kaboom! Similar explosions have happened around the country, so stay safe, little cookers, and for God's sake use the common sense you were born with and don't smoke in the presence of highly flammable gases.

Because Ear Wax is so potent, there have also been a few reports of people freaking out after smoking it, especially the first time. Apparently, the hallucinogenic properties of cannabis are intensified with the high THC content, and the high lasts much longer than usual, so some people end up tripping balls in the worst way. But like any other drug, it's about knowing your limits and using in moderation. Keep in mind that, medically, Ear Wax is used for those with extreme symptoms or a high tolerance to bud, so treat it accordingly and with respect.

INDEX

PICTURE CREDITS

All images are copyright their respective copyright holders and are shown here for historical and review purposes. Every effort has been made to credit the copyright holders, artists and/or studios/publishers whose work has been reproduced in these pages. We apologize for any omissions, which will be corrected in future editions, but must hereby disclaim any liability.

© Roman Sigaev *p2* / © Hein Nouwens *p9* / © Atomazul *p14* / © Daniel J. Rao *p18* / *Marijuana Girl* © 1951 Universal Publishing, New York *p21* / *Marihuana* © 1941 Detective Fiction Weekly, Dell Publishing *p31* / © Featureflash *p34* / Library of Congress, Washington D.C. *p38* / © Lucian Coman *p54* / © aastock *p60* / © Carl Van Vechten, Library of Congress, Washington D.C. *p66* / © Eldad Carin *p75* / *Junkie: Confessions of an Unredeemed Drug Addict* © Ace Books, New York *p88* / © Steven Bostock *p93*